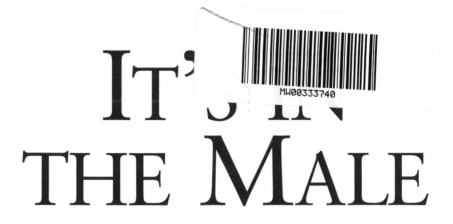

IT'S IN THE MALE

Everyone's Guide to Men's Health

From Infertility to Impotency

and

Testosterone to Prostate Disease

Jon L. Pryor, M.D., and Stacy Glass, R.N.

Minneapolis • Appladay Press • 2000

Illustrations: David J. Mottet

Cover and Page Design: Carbon*Creative*.com

For ordering or information:

1-877-813-4513

www.appladaypress.com

Library of Congress Catalog Number: 190946

ISBN: 0-9678272-0-5

Manufactured in the United States of America

10 9 8 7 6 5 4 3 2 1

In Memory of Bill, our friend,
who died of prostate cancer
on the eve of this book's publication.

Contents

Preface

If you take a tour of the local bookstore, you cannot help but notice all the health books, especially on women's health. The classic *Our Bodies, Ourselves*, published first in 1973, started a whole field of writing on women's health. But virtually absent from the shelves are books on men's health. Recently a few books have dealt with prostate cancer, and a book from the editors of *Men's Health* magazine is a welcome addition. But one would think half the books on health would be for men.

Are men so healthy they don't need information on men's health? Hardly. In fact, many serious health issues relatively unique to males affect the quality and length of their lives. These issues start at birth and continue throughout a man's life.

Do we circumcise our baby boy? When and how does a male do testicular self-examinations? What can a man do when he and his partner have difficulty conceiving a child? After he has children, should he "go under the knife" for a vasectomy? Does male menopause really exist? What can a guy do about impotency or premature ejaculation? How often should men have prostate exams, and what are the implications of prostate cancer? The problems are common. For example, nearly 10 percent of all men are infertile, 20 million men in the United States are impotent, and prostate cancer is the number-one cancer diagnosed in men!

Men's health issues are often difficult to talk about. A guy just does not like to call his doctor's office and ask a nurse or secretary to schedule an appointment regarding impotency. Men get together to play golf and talk about the local sports' teams but usually do not shoot the breeze about their prostates. And parents have a hard time teaching their boys how to do testicular self-examinations.

But men and women do need to know about these things. Knowledge of men's health issues can improve lives, even save them. So if you are a man, or a woman who knows a man, this book is for you. We speak matter-of-factly about issues that many people find difficult to talk or even think about. But we hold nothing back just because it might be embarrassing.

This is not, however, an unabridged edition of everything one could possibly want to know about men. We wanted to keep it under a thousand pages! But it does provide the essentials on some common topics and problems that affect virtually all men.

We have devoted our lives to men's health and hope that our work enlightens and educates all of our readers. But while we want to share our knowledge and stories with you, no one knows it all (we don't!), and everyone has a story to tell. If you have a different perspective, an experience to share, or an area you'd like to know more about, please let us know so that we can include it in future editions. Write us at: Center for Men's Health and Infertility, Department of Urologic Surgery, 420 Delaware St. SE, PO Box 394 FUMC, Minneapolis MN 55455; or Appladay Press, Box 1152, Minnetonka, MN 55345; or on the internet at www.appladaypress.com.

How to Use This Book

Read it; you'll like it. This book is like a consumer guide. It provides lots of information important on men's health. It suggests ways that men can stay healthy and what to do if a problem arises. And it does so in a simple and entertaining way. Necessary medical terms are italicized upon their first appearance. More elaborate definitions of these words appear in the glossary (Appendix 3). No book, however, can substitute for a good healthcare provider. If you have a problem, see your physician, but remember what you learn here. The more you know about men's health, the better the care you will get.

Acknowledgments

We are indebted to many people who helped us write this book. To all the teachers and professors who gave us a foundation of knowledge, particularly Drs. Stuart Howards and Terry Turner at the University of Virginia and Dr. David Hamilton at the University of Minnesota. To our colleges, the University of Minnesota Medical School, and the Fairview University Medical Center, who supported us in so many different ways.

To our friends and family who read through and commented on numerous drafts of this book: Roy Anderson, Jim Anway, Joe Deuhs, Bruce Glass, Elizabeth Boo Neuberger, Laurie Pryor, Thomas Pryor, Dan J. Unger-Weiss, and Andrew Van Bergen, M.D. To all the specialists in medicine who commented on and verified the accuracy of specific chapters: Drs. Michael Pergament, Timothy Schacker, Marcia Shew, Jackson E. Fowler Jr., Reginald C. Bruskewitz, William Utz, Leslie Rainwater, Cesar Ercole, Maria Hordinsky, Eli Coleman, Bruce Redmon, and Jeff Balke.

To David J. Mottet, our superb illustrator. To our patients, who trust us and help us to learn as we help them. And finally, to our families, who put up with so much as we immersed ourselves in our writing. To all of you, many, many thanks!

1

Foreskin
Circumcision, penile cancer, and controversies

It's hard to believe something as simple as foreskin could be so controversial. Many in the medical field and the general public firmly believe circumcision should not be performed. Some even belong to societies for the preservation of foreskin. But when today's baby boomers were infants, the removal of foreskin was nearly universal. Here we explain what foreskin is, the process of circumcision, and the pros and cons of this procedure.

Anatomy

The end or head of the penis is called the *glans*. The glans is where the opening of the urethra (the tube through which a male urinates) is located. When a baby boy is born, the foreskin covers the glans so that the head of the penis cannot be seen.

The Controversy

Nearly 80 percent of all men in the United States are circumcised. In some religions, such as Judaism, circumcision is virtually universal. Probably the main reason for circumcision is simply that parents want it for their sons. Their reasons, apart from religion, typically include concerns such as "better hygiene," "we don't know anyone who isn't circumcised," and "we want him to look like his father."

Potential health benefits of circumcision include the prevention of penile cancer. Cancer of the penis can be fatal, and treating this cancer often involves removing a portion of the penis. Cancer of the penis in areas of Africa and Asia, where circumcision is uncommon, accounts for 10 to 20 percent of all cancers in men. In contrast, penile cancer constitutes approximately 1 percent of all cancers in men within the United States.

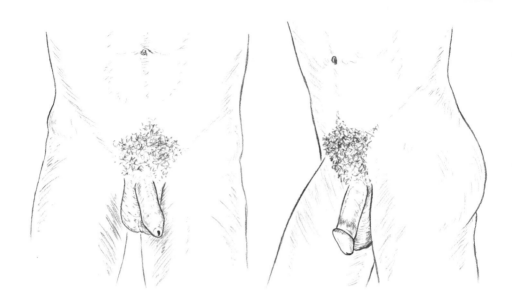

Left, an uncircumcised penis. Right, a circumcised penis. Notice that the foreskin of the uncircumcised penis covers the glans so it cannot be seen.

Males circumcised around the time of puberty face a decreased incidence of penile cancer. But in groups, including the Jewish population, who remove foreskin at birth, penile cancer is almost unknown. This is pretty convincing evidence that new-born circumcision prevents penile cancer. But circumcision in an adult male offers no protection from penile cancer.

How does circumcision help prevent penile cancer? Cleaning a circumcised penis is slightly easier than cleaning an uncircumcised one. A collection of sloughed skin and bacteria (*smegma*), which is white and cheeselike, can collect under the fore-skin of an uncircumcised penis. Smegma may be carcinogenic. So an uncircumcised male should retract the foreskin and clean the head of the penis on a daily basis. Smegma does not accumulate on a circumcised penis, so no hygiene other than routine baths or showers is necessary.

Some studies suggest that circumcision decreases the chances of a child getting a urinary tract infection. Lower rates of sexually transmitted diseases such as herpes and venereal warts (like warts on a finger, but these are warts on the penis) occur in the circumcised male as compared to the uncircumcised male.

The primary reason not to have circumcision is that it is not necessary. Uncircumcised men who pull back the foreskin and clean the penis on a routine basis probably face no increased chance of getting penile cancer. With good sexual practices such as wearing a condom, the chances of getting herpes or other sexually transmitted diseases should not be any different in the uncircumcised man than those in the circumcised man. Maybe the best reason not to circumcise is that some people claim an uncircumcised man has increased sensation in the head of the penis, which makes sex more pleasurable.

So should a baby be circumcised or not? There is no right answer. As previously stated, most newborns are probably circumcised out of tradition: the father is circumcised and therefore the son is too. Parents who choose circumcision may do so without guilt. But circumcision is not medically necessary. If problems with foreskin develop in the future, circumcision can be done at that time.

The debate on circumcision tends to be cyclical. Back in the 1960s and 1970s, nearly all baby boys in the United States were circumcised. In one school I (J.P.) attended, only one boy was not. We were too young even to know what foreskin was, and most of us had seen the heads of circumcised penises only. So many of us thought this individual had a crippling disease, and some of us shunned him.

In 1975, the American Academy of Pediatrics declared that circumcision is totally unnecessary. In 1989, it slightly reversed that declaration, saying there might be medical reasons for performing a circumcision. If you think the medical world is a little schizophrenic on this issue, you are correct. Currently there are no particular leanings one way or another. Like many things in life, there is no clear-cut answer that is valid for everyone. Undoubtedly, the debate will continue.

Circumcision, the Procedure

A newborn boy may be circumcised if he is delivered at around 40 weeks, is healthy, big enough, and has no problems with his penis. If the baby does not pee out of the end of his penis or something appears to be wrong with the penis, the opening of the penis may be in the wrong place. Parents and the pediatrician should check it out. If the opening is abnormal, circumcision should not be done as the foreskin can be used later, like a skin graft, to fix the penis.

If both baby and penis look good, circumcision usually is performed before the newborn leaves the hospital. The child is restrained, and the penis is cleaned. An anesthetic should be injected around the penis to lessen pain. In the past, anesthetics were uncommon because physicians believed newborns did not feel pain. We believe, after doing many of these procedures, that their crying indicates babies do feel pain and that an anesthetic should be given.

After the penis is numbed, the physician retracts the foreskin and puts a shield, called a bell, around the head of the penis. Then the surgeon clamps the foreskin to squish the excess foreskin where it meets the bell. This excess foreskin is cut off, and the bell and clamp are removed. Usually, no stitching is necessary. Antiseptic ointment or petroleum jelly is applied, then reapplied several times a day during diaper changes until the wound is completely healed, about one week after circumcision. This care helps prevent infection and keeps the circumcised area from sticking to the diaper.

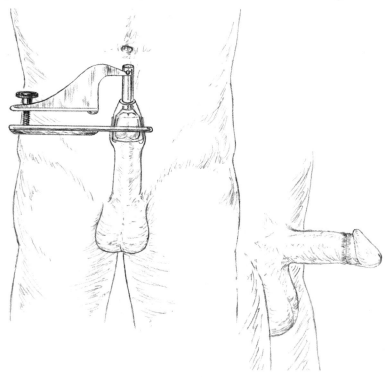

At left a bell protects the head of the penis during circumcision of a newborn. At right is the result—a circumcised penis.

Complications from circumcision include the removal of too much or too little foreskin. Also, the edges of the skin crimped by the bell and clamp may separate. If something looks abnormal or if complications occur, parents should take their child to a pediatric urologist for further inspection of the penis and possible treatment.

Bells are not made large enough for the circumcision of boys beyond six months of age, so a different procedure is used for them. A general anesthetic is given to boys from six months to teenage years so that they will sleep through circumcision. For adults, the penis is numbed with a local anesthetic. Then an incision is made around the foreskin both on the outside of the penis and the inside of the foreskin. This band of excess foreskin is then cut off, leaving two edges of skin to be stitched together. The procedure takes about 15 to 30 minutes, and the patient goes home the same day. As with any surgical procedure, there is a slight risk of infection or bleeding.

Foreskin Problems

An uncircumcised man may be subject to *phimosis*. With this condition the foreskin cannot be retracted, so the head of the penis (glans) never sees the light of day. Phimosis makes cleaning the head of the penis difficult—a setup for infection of the glans and foreskin. Phimosis may cause the head of the penis to be sore especially during intercourse, which is a bad time to be hurting. Severe phimosis may make urination difficult. The best treatment for persistent phimosis is circumcision.

Phimosis is normal for baby boys. But by five years of age almost all uncircumcised boys have retractable foreskin.

The condition opposite phimosis is *paraphimosis*. Remember learning in kindergarten to put everything back where you found it? When the foreskin is retracted for whatever reason, eventually it must go back over the head of the penis. If not, the foreskin may tighten, swell, and become painful making it difficult to pull back at all. Firm and constant pressure, along with a little lubrication, usually works to get the foreskin back over the head of the penis. A physician experienced with these conditions may be required. If the foreskin cannot be brought back over the head of the penis, circumcision is needed.

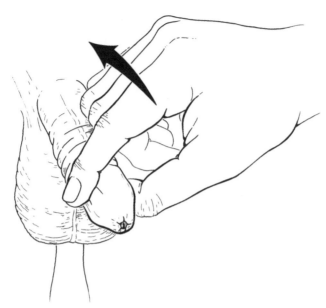

With phimosis, the foreskin cannot be retracted to expose the head of the penis.

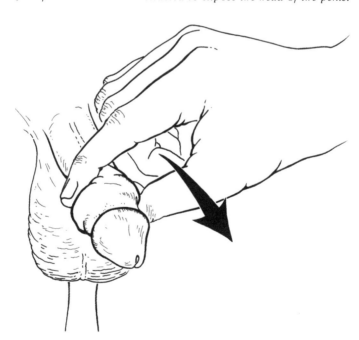

With paraphimosis, the opposite of phimosis, the foreskin cannot be pulled back to cover the head of the penis. This swelling may occur if the foreskin is left in the retracted position.

Another condition, more common in the uncircumcised than the circumcised man, is *balanitis*. With this condition, the head of the penis and the foreskin become infected, swollen, painful, and red. Topical antiseptic agents rubbed on the infected area will kill the bacteria. In severe cases, oral antibiotics are recommended. If the inflamed foreskin does not improve or infection occurs frequently, circumcision probably is indicated.

Finally, numerous sores, bumps, or lumps may occur on the foreskin. Some of these indicate sexually transmitted disease. Others are just little areas of infection that come and go on their own. Still others may be penile cancer. If a new sore or lump appears on the penis, the man should see a doctor. Often the initial diagnosis is infection or inflammation with a remedy of steroid cream or antiseptic to make the sore go away. If the sore doesn't get better or the physician cannot identify the sore or lump, a second opinion or biopsy is in order.

A biopsy is a relatively simple procedure usually done in a clinic. A sample from the lump is extracted for examination under a microscope, so that an exact diagnosis can be made. Men should not avoid checking something out for fear they have penile cancer. With early detection, the cancer may be removed and the penis saved. As with all cancers, the goal is to catch it early before it progresses.

The Bottom Line

- Having foreskin is normal. Males are born with it. Foreskin is not an abnormal condition.

- Medical reasons for circumcision include decreased chances of urinary tract infections in baby boys and of sexually transmitted diseases later in life. The incidence of penile cancer is rare in men circumcised as infants.

- With proper hygiene, which includes retracting the foreskin and washing the penile area on a daily basis, circumcision usually is not necessary.

- If you choose circumcision for your son, make that decision without guilt.

- When you retract the foreskin to clean the head of the penis, to urinate, or for whatever reason, be sure to put it back. Otherwise paraphimosis may develop.

- If new sores or lumps develop on the penis, seek medical attention. Odds are, they can be easily treated. Ignoring a sore or lump is dangerous.

2

Good Sexual Health
From infancy to adulthood

Sexual health involves religions, cultures, individual beliefs, and values. Obviously, people can sincerely disagree about it. But there are some basic principles that every male should understand.

Erections

Males start having erections the day they are born. Most would like to continue having them until the day they die. Erections often occur at night (nocturnal erections). They also happen intermittently throughout the day. Sometimes they occur with sexual thoughts or stimulation; other times they happen on their own. Think of erections as a completely normal and healthy aspect of human life, just like breathing. In fact, that old adage "use it or lose it" really does apply to erections. The experts now think men "need" erections to get oxygen to the penis and keep its tissue healthy. Without nighttime and daily erections, the penis would not get the oxygen it needs, and some of its healthy tissue could turn into scar tissue.

Puberty

Everyone wants to be young, but we doubt many would jump at the chance to go through puberty again. Generally, boys have little change in their penises or testicles from birth to the beginning of puberty. Puberty for males usually starts somewhere around the age of 12 or 13 and lasts several years. Puberty that begins before age nine may indicate a hormonal problem called precocious puberty. It can be treated. When the early physical changes of puberty are not present by age 14, this also may indicate a hormonal problem. In either case have it evaluated.

Puberty is usually triggered by a surge of *testosterone* that causes the testicles and penis to grow, the scrotal skin to thicken and "redden," and wrinkles called *rugae* to develop in the scrotum. In other areas of the body, testosterone causes the development of *secondary sexual characteristics*, such as facial, pubic, and armpit hair growth and a deepening of the voice.

Try to remember what it's like going through puberty. It is a time of tremendous social as well as physical change. *Hormones* rage and sexual awareness begins. This is a good time for the adolescent to read about puberty and sexuality. If a friend tells you something that sounds strange, check it out from a more reputable source—a book, parents, teachers, or doctors. For example, when I (J.P.) was a teenager, a friend told me that a man gets only so many erections in his lifetime, and when they are used up, he is impotent. I believed this fallacy until medical school. Then I learned impotency has nothing to do with the number of erections a guy had when he was younger. What a relief!

Parents and teenagers should view puberty as a normal process. Adolescent sons will have legitimate questions and concerns about sexuality and related topics. These questions are not strange or perverted but completely normal for adolescents. Encourage them. Open communication is certainly the best way to guide your son to a healthy sexual experience for life. If a parent or child feels communication is difficult or lacking on these issues, a nurse, physician, or other healthcare worker may be a good resource. Even experts on sex like us find talking to our children about these issues difficult. It's amazing how much easier it is to speak to teenagers other than our own about sex. If we feel this way, many other parents must share this uneasiness. So consider outside advice and counseling an acceptable alternative to parent-son discussions about sexuality.

Masturbation

We believe most males masturbate. Typically, masturbation begins around the onset of puberty. Tremendous guilt may be associated with masturbation. This guilt may be self-imposed, spread by friends, perpetrated by family, or taught by religion. Since virtually all males masturbate, we feel it is natural and should not cause guilt.

Further, masturbation does not necessarily stop after a man has established sexual relations with a partner. Most men continue to masturbate throughout their sexual lives, even after marriage. Though the frequency may decrease once a man starts to have sex with a partner or as he ages, masturbation tends to be a part of a man's life forever. This does not mean a man loves his partner less or does not enjoy intercourse or other sexual relations with his partner. Men may continue to masturbate because of sexual urges or out of habit.

Though masturbation is usually not a big deal, it can be a problem if done at the wrong time or in the wrong place (for example, the library is not a good place to do it). It also may be a problem for partners who "should" be having sex with each other but don't because the guy masturbates so frequently he has no further desire. This can affect a relationship!

Intercourse, Sexual Diseases, and Condoms, Condoms, Condoms

When a guy has intercourse, he should wear a condom! Okay, maybe he should not wear one if he and his partner are trying to have a baby. But if you want to prevent a pregnancy and the spread of sexually transmitted diseases (STDs), condoms are great.

A tremendous number of STDs lie in wait out there. Many of these diseases have no symptoms and so go undetected. Some, like chlamydia and gonorrhea, are relatively easy to treat. Genital herpes stays with a man forever and, if passed on to a woman who becomes pregnant, can affect the fetus or the baby when she delivers. Others, like venereal warts, are not only unsightly but ultimately can lead to cervical cancer in the female partner. Still others, like HIV, kill.

Crabs (genital lice), though one of the less-severe STDs, can spread through a college dormitory like wildfire. People may be infested through intercourse or by sitting on a contaminated bed. Crabs are difficult to see, but anyone who has uncontrollable itching in the groin and notices little bugs or white spots in the pubic hair probably has crabs. Luckily, you can get rid of these pesky critters with an over-the-counter lice shampoo and a good washing of contaminated bedding and clothes. Occasionally, a prescription is necessary.

Human papilloma virus (HPV or genital warts) looks like tiny cauliflower or little bumps on the genitals. It can be visible on the penis or so small you cannot see it. Sometimes the bumps are inside the urethra (the tube in the penis that urine passes through). These urethral warts can cause burning during urination or blood in the urine. In females, HPV is even more difficult to detect because it can be hidden in the vagina.

If there are a few warts and all are visible (that is, they are not in the urethra), a solution called podophyllin may be applied. Podophyllin will cure about half of all warts. Some new creams for application, as well as some new medications for injection into warts, stimulate a patient's immune system (*white blood cells*) to attack warts. If these medications do not work or if there are warts in the urethra, a physician can burn them off with a laser. Be persistent in getting rid of genital warts. If left untreated, they may become infected. And with time, some warts cause cervical cancer in women (HPV is said to be the number-one cause of cervical cancer) or penile cancer in men.

Chlamydia is an infection caused by a bacteria-like organism that attacks the lining of the urethra and reproductive organs such as the *epididymis*. Some men with chlamydia have no symptoms. Others have frequency problems, pain with urination, or a clear or white discharge from the end of the penis. To determine whether chlamydia is present, a small cotton swab is inserted into the urethra, then sent for special testing. Chlamydia is treated with antibiotics. If left untreated, an infection may get worse or even cause infertility.

Gonorrhea (also gonococcus or GC for short) is similar to chlamydia in symptoms, but the symptoms usually are more obvious. There is yellow discharge at the end of the urethra. To determine whether someone has GC, a small cotton swab is inserted into the urethra (the same as for chlamydia), and special tests are done on the swab. If a man has GC, both he and his partner need antibiotics. If gonorrhea is left untreated, a severe infection of the entire genital system can occur. And again, fertility problems may result from the scar tissue that forms from the extensive infection. Therefore, early detection and treatment for all STDs is important.

Genital herpes lives with you forever. The sores or lesions that occur with this type of herpes can occur anywhere on the genitals. The sores are often painful. They remain for two to three weeks and then go away, but they will reoccur periodically, from one to several times a year, for the rest of your life. Medications such as acyclovir can help relieve symptoms and limit the outbreak of sores. When the sores are present, herpes can be transferred to another person through sexual contact. But herpes virus can also be spread when there are no warning signs. A person infected with herpes may spread the virus *without* a sore—just another reason to practice safe sex.

One of the most deadly and most-talked-about diseases is acquired immune deficiency syndrome (AIDS). AIDS is caused by a virus called human immunodeficiency virus (HIV). HIV can be transmitted through blood, *semen*, vaginal fluids, or breast milk. HIV has to be spread through an opening in the skin or through mucous membranes such as the vagina, rectum, or mouth. For example, HIV in semen can be transmitted to a woman through a sore in the vagina or by oral sex. Likewise, someone stuck with a contaminated needle can become infected. But it is virtually impossible to get HIV by shaking hands or even kissing someone with HIV. The late Princess of Wales, Diana, made a big point of touching children and adults with HIV to show the world we need not avoid or fear contact with those who have HIV.

Blood tests can determine whether a person has HIV. Anyone who has HIV when tested is likely to develop AIDS. Some will develop AIDS soon; in others it may take many years. AIDS turns off the body's ability to fight disease. Symptoms of AIDS are fever, fatigue, night sweats, enlarged *lymph nodes*, loss of appetite, unexplained weight loss, difficulty breathing, and a hacking cough. Death usually occurs from infections or cancers that the body can no longer fight off.

Treatment involves a course of medication to stop the virus from multiplying and dealing with illnesses that develop because of AIDS. At the time of this writing, there is no cure for AIDS, but many new medications are emerging to help prolong life. Despite these new medications, we all must think prevention, push for more research, and hope for a cure. A World Health Organization report at the end of 1997 showed that 16,000 people contract HIV every day, nearly double previous estimates. Worldwide, about 30 million people are HIV-positive.

As you can see, signs and symptoms vary from one sexually transmitted disease to another. If you or your partner develop burning with urination, pain with *ejaculation* or intercourse, sores or warts on the penis or vaginal area, an unusual penile or vaginal discharge, and/or itching, see a healthcare professional! If only one partner is treated and sex is resumed, the STD can spread back and forth again between the partners.

This book is dedicated to preventive medicine: how do we stay healthy? With that in mind, the best way for a sexually active man to avoid STDs is to wear a condom. Latex condoms are better than those made from animal skin for preventing the spread of disease by the transmission of viruses and bacteria. Using a condom gives the added benefit of preventing unwanted pregnancies. Still another benefit is that the dulling of sensation in the penis may allow the guy better control of the timing of ejaculation.

Though condoms are great—they are one sign of a responsible man—they are not perfect. Viruses can penetrate them or a condom may break or slip off. If the condom is used improperly, semen may leak around it. Some people are allergic to latex condoms. This would appear as pain, itching, and redness on the penis or around the vagina after using a latex condom. Latex allergies are rare, but if you are allergic, use a nonlatex or animal-skin condom instead.

Penile Trauma

A rigid penis can actually bend and break. This is called a *fractured penis*. Of course, the penis has no bone to break, but the tissue can tear. A fractured penis may result from bending the penis during masturbation. Or it may occur during vigorous intercourse if the penis hits the pelvis bone of the partner and it bends too much. Sharp pain and swelling are the result. Though a fractured penis is rare, it does require prompt medical attention. Surgical treatment is necessary to repair the torn tissues and prevent future problems with erections.

Penises sometimes end up in strange places such as vacuum cleaners or bottles, or adorned with ornaments such as rings or jewelry. In general, such habitats are not good for the penis, which may become infected, swollen, torn, or physically beaten up. Masturbation is great, but placing your penis in these situations may lead to medical problems as well as embarrassment. Just imagine going to your local emergency room with a vacuum cleaner attached to your penis!

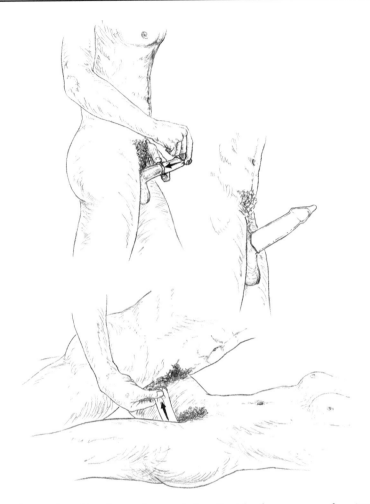

Correct use of a condom: Put the condom on before foreplay because sexual excitement may cause sperm to come outside the penis long before ejaculation. At top, hold the tip to squeeze out air and leave space for semen to collect after ejaculation. Roll the condom all the way down to the pubic hair at the base of the penis. At bottom, hold the condom in place after intercourse so it comes out with the penis and does not spill or leak. Do this right after ejaculation, while the penis is still hard. Discard the condom; do not use it again.

What Should and Should Not Come Out of the Penis

Besides pleasure, lots of different things come from the penis. To be precise, lots of things come out of the urethra, the tube that urine goes through. With sexual stimulation, a clear fluid appears at the end of the urethra. Glands inside the urethra produce this clear lubricant that helps with penetration during sex. Though the fluid is not "ejaculate," it may contain some sperm, as well as any of the STDs. So put the condom on early, during foreplay, if you are trying to prevent a pregnancy or the spread of STDs.

With ejaculation, about one-half to one full teaspoon of fluid, called *semen*, comes from the urethra. A common misconception is that semen and sperm are the same. Semen is both fluid and sperm. Only a small amount of semen, about 1 percent, is actually sperm. The rest of semen is fluid, primarily from the prostate and *seminal vesicles*. The seminal vesicles are glands, close to the bladder, that connect with the urethra. Semen has a musty odor, but its odor as well as its appearance may change with diet, frequency of ejaculation, and age.

Blood may come out of the urethra, too. Blood visible in the urine is called *gross hematuria* (gross because the blood can be seen, not because it is nasty). Gross hematuria may be caused by cancer of the kidney or bladder, an enlarged prostate (see chapter 10, on benign prostatic hyperplasia), or a urinary tract infection. Blood that appears as a discharge or secretion from the urethra, but that is not visible in the urine, often shows up as a bloodstain on underwear. This blood may also be from cancer (often of the prostate or bladder, less often of the kidney), an enlarged prostate, an infection, or trauma to the penis. If a man has gross hematuria or a bloody urethral discharge, he should see his physician. Ignoring the warning signs of blood in urine or urethral discharge is dangerous. In most cases whatever is causing the bleeding, even if it happens to be cancer, can be treated successfully.

Sometimes there is blood in the ejaculate, which is called *hematospermia*. Physicians cannot always explain why the blood appears, but usually it is nothing to worry about. It often goes away after one or two ejaculations. If the blood persists, however, see your physician.

Finally, after a bowel movement, a urethral discharge similar to ejaculate but smaller in amount may occur. This happens because the stool passes the prostate and expresses prostatic fluids into the urethra. This is similar to the fluid expressed by the *prostatic massage* that physicians sometimes use to check for infection in the prostate. Prostatic massages are not frequent, but bowel movements are. The resulting urethral discharge is normal.

Sexual Identity: A Few Thoughts on Bisexuality

Some people believe everyone can be classified as strictly heterosexual or homosexual. That is a myth. Some people may fit in one of these two categories, but there's a lot in between. Some would label everything between heterosexual and homosexual as bisexual, but even this gets confusing. One expert, for example, has said that about 20 percent of the men who identify themselves as homosexual have had sex with a woman. Does this mean they are bisexual? And what about all the men who are bisexual in thought, fantasy, or emotional attachment, but strictly heterosexual in behavior? Are they bisexual or heterosexual?

Since we cannot read one another's thoughts and we all think and fantasize about many different things, we usually attach labels of sexuality to behavior. But many people have the potential for bisexuality. Wherever you end up on the spectrum of sexual identity, choose a healthy sexual life.

The Bottom Line

- Masturbation is natural—for teenagers, for adults, for happily married senior citizens. Men and women who recognize this will feel comfortable about masturbation. Discussing issues of sexuality—with parents, with children, with medical personnel, or with other trusted people—is healthy. Sex is everywhere in our society, and ignoring it will not make it go away. Frequent communication about questions and concerns can lead to safer and more enjoyable sexual lifestyles.

- Unless you've been in a monogamous relationship for several years or you and your partner are trying to conceive, always use condoms during sexual intercourse. Sexually transmitted diseases occur even in the elderly.

- If you have symptoms of a sexually transmitted disease, seek prompt medical attention. If only one partner seeks treatment, the other partner may spread the disease to others or reinfect the one treated.

- Blood in the urine or in a urethral discharge may be a warning sign of cancer or infection. Check it out with a physician.

3

The Testicle
From lumps and bumps to pain

Unlike ovaries (the internal female reproductive organs), testicles are located outside the male body in a sac called the *scrotum*. As one woman has informed us, the testicles and scrotum do not hang out to be admired for their beauty. Rather, the testicles must be in the scrotum, away from the body, so that sperm can develop at the proper temperature. For sperm, this is cooler than normal body temperature.

The external placement is both a blessing and a curse. It allows the testicle to be inspected so that testicular cancer can be detected early and treated successfully. But the testicle makes a great target for softballs, bike bars, and knees. Learning what is in the scrotum and how to take good care of the testicles is essential to men's health.

Anatomy

The skin that covers the testicles is called the scrotum. Before birth, testicles reside in the abdomen. As the fetus develops, the testicles usually descend into the scrotum. Once inside the scrotum, the left testicle often hangs a little lower than the right. The left testicle not only hangs a little lower, but it is also a little smaller than the right. The difference, however, is subtle, and to most men the testicles appear to be the same size. The average adult testicle is one-and-a-half to two inches long and an inch wide.

The testicles are egg-shaped structures with two primary purposes: to develop sperm, also called *germ cells*, and to produce testosterone, a male hormone. Although many men believe testosterone comes from the penis, the testicles produce 95 percent of a man's testosterone.

Sperm develop from cells called *spermatogonia*, within long, thin tubes called *seminiferous tubules*. As spermatogonia mature, they divide into more advanced germ

18

cells called *spermatocytes*. Most germ cells are at the spermatogonia or early spermatocyte stage when a baby boy is born. The germ cells stay at these stages until the boy reaches puberty. Then they develop into more advanced germ cells called *spermatids*. The spermatids mature and eventually are released from the seminiferous tubules. At this stage they are *spermatozoa* or sperm.

From the testicle the sperm travel through a single, highly coiled tube behind the testicle called the epididymis. The *epididymis* looks like angel-hair pasta except that it is much smaller and tightly coiled. Uncoiled, the epididymis would be about five yards long. The sperm start their journey at the head of the epididymis (called the *caput* epididymis) located at the top of the testicle. As sperm travel down the epididymal tube, they mature and become more capable of fertilizing the female's egg.

Sperm are stored in the tail of the epididymis (called the *cauda* epididymis) until they are ejaculated. Ejaculation pushes them through a tube connected to the epididymis called the *vas deferens*, then expels them through the ejaculatory duct in the prostate. They mix with fluid from the prostate and structures around it, then are forced out the urethra during ejaculation.

The whole process of sperm development from spermatogonia until ejaculation takes three months. So if you have a fever or are exposed to a toxic material that affects developing sperm, three months may pass before the sperm count goes down (see chapter 5, on infertility).

Though seminiferous tubules and sperm cells make up most of the volume of the testis, the *Leydig cells*, also in the testis, make testosterone, which is secreted into the bloodstream. Testosterone is important for developing secondary sexual characteristics—a deeper voice, beard, pubic hair, sexual drive, and muscle. Testosterone is also important to the development of sperm. Without it, sperm and other substances associated with reproduction would not develop.

The Undescended Testicle

In about one-third of premature male infants and 3 percent of newborns, the testicles do not descend normally. Usually with a little time and growth, the testicle comes down on its own during the first year of life. A testicle that does not come down is called an undescended testicle or *cryptorchidism*. Pediatricians routinely check for cryptorchidism during infant exams.

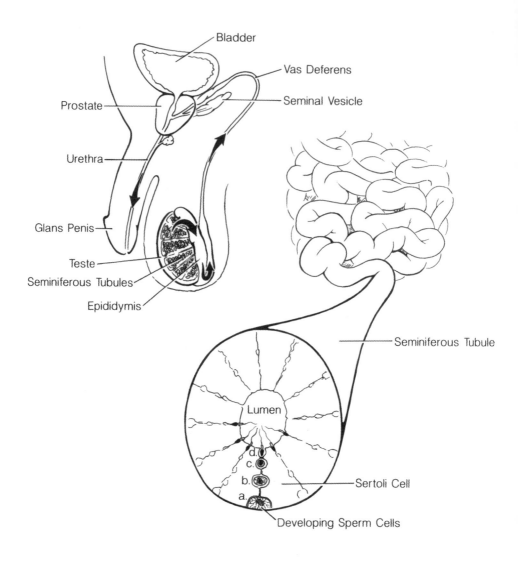

At top, sperm develop in the seminiferous tubules within the testicle. At bottom, the sperm start as spermatogonia (a) at the outside edge of the seminiferous tubule. As they develop through the stages of spermatocyte (b) to spermatid (c), they move towards the center of the seminiferous tubule to where there is a space or lumen. The sperm (d) are then released into the lumen to travel to the epididymis, where they are stored until ejaculation.

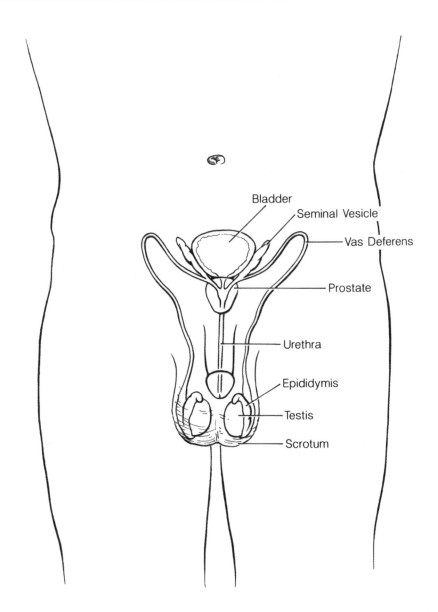

Bladder

Seminal Vesicle

Vas Deferens

Prostate

Urethra

Epididymis

Testis

Scrotum

The testicles lie within a sac called the scrotum. After sperm develop in the testicle, they are stored in the epididymis behind each testicle. Ejaculation pushes the sperm through the vas deferens to the ejaculatory duct within the prostate. Here the sperm mix with fluids from the prostate and seminal vesicles before coming out the urethra. It's quite a journey.

Sometimes the testicle can be felt in the upper scrotum and pulled down to the bottom of the scrotum. This is a condition called a *retractile* testis. In general, it is nothing to worry about. Often the testicle will move to the bottom of the scrotum as the child develops and goes through puberty. But if the testicle cannot be brought to the bottom of the scrotum, this mild form of cryptorchidism should prompt further evaluation.

Sometimes medications can help the testicle descend. But if a testicle is not descended by the first birthday, surgery is in order. The testicle must be brought into the scrotum so that it is cool enough for sperm to develop. The surgical procedure for bringing the testicle down into the scrotum is called *orchiopexy*. A pediatric urologist or pediatric surgeon usually performs it. A relatively simple procedure when performed by an experienced surgeon, it is done on an outpatient basis.

Males with a history of undescended testicles have a slightly higher chance of developing testicular cancer, even when the testicle is brought down into the scrotum. Notice we said "slightly higher." Most guys who have had an undescended testicle will *not* develop testicular cancer. But if the testicle is brought down, at least you can check it on a regular basis (do a testicular self-exam) to detect any cancer early. Read on.

Testicular Self-Examination and Testicular Cancer

Testicular cancer is one of the most common cancers in young men. It affects about 5,000 males in the United States each year. This cancer tends to affect men from age 15 to 35, but it can occur in babies as well as in older men.

Testicular cancer usually shows up as a painless lump or mass on the testicle. This is important: you detect the cancer not by pain but by feeling a lump or swelling. If cancer is suspected, a urologist will explore the testicle. If it appears cancerous, the urologist will remove the testicle through an incision in the area of the upper thigh. Additional treatment may include radiation therapy for certain types of testicular cancer (seminoma), surgery to remove lymph nodes in the abdomen to prevent spread, and chemotherapy. The cure rate is very high, especially if you catch the cancer early. Even if the cancer has spread, the cure rate with modern chemotherapy is high. If a man with testicular cancer (or any cancer for that matter) is going to get radiation or chemotherapy, he should seriously consider freezing and banking his sperm before the treatment starts. This is because radiation or chemotherapy can damage the testicle, making the man infertile. Thinking about fertility is difficult when cancer is on the mind, but many men have thanked us afterwards for encouraging them to bank sperm before getting radiation or chemotherapy.

Testicular cancers also may develop in children. Though these are different from the cancers that develop in teenagers or men, the treatment options are similar. As with most diseases, the worst thing you can do with testicular cancer is to ignore it. We recently had several patients who felt something abnormal but, from fear or denial, failed to have it checked out. Just about the only way to die from testicular cancer is to pretend it isn't there. So if you have any question about something in the scrotum, ask your physician to check it out.

Just as women should do routine self-exams on their breasts, men should do routine testicular exams to screen for cancer. The age to start checking the testicle for masses is at puberty or about age 15. Boys and men should check their testicles about once a month.

The scrotum is looser and the testicles easier to feel in a warm environment such as in the shower. So the shower may be a convenient place in which to check for lumps or bumps. To do a testicular self-exam, feel carefully with your hand all areas of both left and right testicles. Remember that the epididymis is behind the testicle, and this is a normal structure. The first time you examine yourself things may not feel quite right—this is unfamiliar territory. But after several examinations you will get used to what is normal. Then, if a lump develops, you will notice the difference, and you should promptly see a physician.

Scrotal and Testicular Pain or Great Balls of Fire

Testicular pain may be severe and indicate a need for immediate medical attention or simply be a mild pain of unknown cause. In general, sudden and severe testicular pain should be checked immediately by a doctor.

Sudden and severe testicular pain may be from an infection. An infection of the epididymis is called *epididymitis*, of the testicle *orchitis*, and of the epididymis and testicle *epididymo-orchitis*. These infections frequently develop over several days. The result may be a painful testicle, a burning sensation with urination, and a fever.

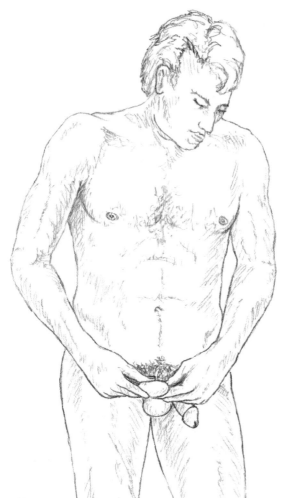

A testicular self-exam.

Epididymitis and epididymo-orchitis are usually treated with antibiotics. They often clear up with this therapy. If a pocket or collection of infection called an *abscess* has developed, surgical draining may be necessary.

On occasion, severe testicular pain comes from a twisted testicle cutting off its own blood supply. This is testicular *torsion*. The pain usually occurs suddenly, sometimes with nausea and vomiting. Testicular torsion is a surgical emergency. The scrotum must be surgically explored immediately and the testicle untwisted. If the blood supply is cut off for too long, the testicle will die and have to be removed.

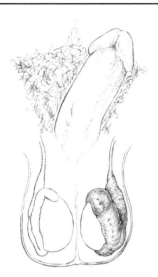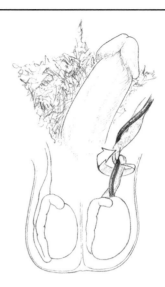

At left is a case of an infection (epididymitis) with an inflamed epididymis. At right is a twisted, or torsed, testicle. This condition is considered an emergency. If it is not fixed quickly, the testicle will die from lack of blood.

Though torsion tends to occur in teenagers and young adults, and epididymitis in older adults, these problems can occur at any age. Distinguishing between torsion and an infection of the testicle is often difficult. If you have severe pain, and no definite diagnosis, the safest thing is a trip to the operating room for an exploration of the scrotum. If the testicle is infected, not twisted, there's no harm done. But if there is torsion, immediate exploration can often save the life of the testicle. Again, the sudden onset of testicular pain in any child, teenager, or adult should be considered an emergency. Seek immediate medical attention.

Slowly developing, mild pain in the testicle is called chronic scrotal pain. It has numerous potential causes. It may result from a mild, long-term infection in the epididymis or prostate, from a *hydrocele*, or from a vasectomy (*post-vasectomy pain syndrome*, see chapter 6). Often an exact cause for chronic scrotal pain is not found.

A man with persistent scrotal pain or discomfort should see his physician for diagnosis and treatment. Rarely can the physician guarantee the pain will go away. For example, *prostatitis* (an infection or inflammation in the prostate gland) can cause pain in the testicle. Antibiotics may take the pain away—or not. Likewise, a *varicocele* (dilated veins of the scrotum) may be detected and treated. The pain should go away, but sometimes it will not.

Chronic scrotal pain is an unpredictable condition, but here are some general rules for treating it. Start conservatively with nonsteroidal anti-inflammatory agents such as aspirin or ibuprofen and wear scrotal support (a jock strap). Try antibiotics if there appears to be an infection. If conservative treatment does not work, surgery is an option when a specific problem is found. For example, if a varicocele is present in the scrotum, a varicocelectomy (surgery to tie off enlarged veins) can be performed. On occasion a patient is so bothered by pain that he wants his testicle removed. Even removing the testicle may not relieve the pain, however, so surgery should be viewed as a last resort. Under no circumstance should an adolescent undergo removal of the testicle or epididymis because of scrotal pain. Only adult males who do not desire children in the furure should consider this option.

Pain that cannot be eliminated is called chronic pain syndrome. For chronic pain, therapies such as psychological counseling, antidepressants (these medications seem to lessen pain), long-term electrical stimulation (transcutaneous electrical nerve stimulation or TENS), and psychological support may help.

Biofeedback—using the mind to control the body—and other coping skills may be useful as well. You can learn about these therapies at a pain clinic. There you will find physicians offering unique treatments to patients with chronic pain of all kinds. Chronic pain syndrome means pain may be a lifelong problem that you'll have to learn to live with.

The Varicocele

One of the more common masses or "funny things" felt in the scrotum is a varicocele. Varicoceles are enlarged veins in the scrotum, like varicose veins in the leg. They often feel like a bag of worms or a squishy tube. A varicocele is most common on the left side (two-thirds of cases). In about one-third of cases, varicoceles are found on both the left and right sides. Rarely are varicoceles just on the right side.

Varicoceles occur in 15 percent of all men. They usually develop with the onset of puberty. The majority of men (about five out of six) have no problem with a varicocele. But about one in six men with a varicocele has problems with fertility and testicular growth.

A varicocele discovered in the smaller testicle of an adolescent, or in an adolescent whose testicles are growing too slowly, should be treated. A varicocele in an adult having problems with fertility also should be treated. Finally, varicoceles associated with scrotal pain can be treated. But as previously discussed, treating the varicocele may not make the pain go away.

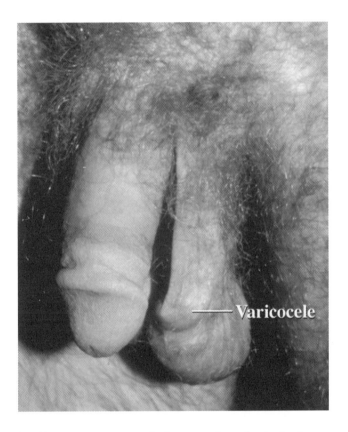

Varicoceles, like varicose veins in the leg, are enlarged veins in the scrotum.

Treating a varicocele involves blocking or obstructing the vein. This can be done by a radiologist, who will implant coils, balloons, or substances that scar the testicular vein. This is called *embolization*. The varicoceles can also be blocked surgically (varicocelectomy) by a urologist, who will tie off the veins in the *inguinal* or groin area or a little higher by the hip. Though it may not sound like it, this is relatively minor surgery easily performed on an outpatient basis.

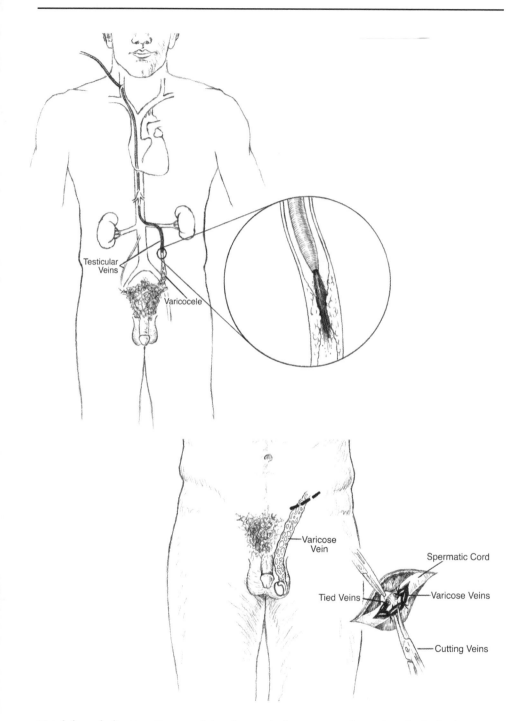

Top left, embolization. Bottom right, the surgical treatment of a varicocele. In both approaches the goal of treatment is to block or obstruct the enlarged veins.

Hydrocele

A hydrocele is a collection of fluid around the testicle. It makes the scrotum look big or swollen. Hydroceles are common and occur in babies as well as men. They may remain small and cause no problem. Other times they become much larger and more painful. We have seen some as large as footballs. Though not life-threatening, hydroceles can be bothersome, and rarely do they go away on their own. A bothersome one can be treated relatively easily by surgically removing the sac that contains the fluid.

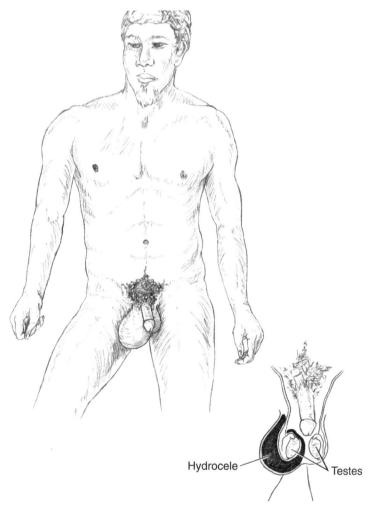

A hydrocele in the right scrotum makes this man appear to have a big right testicle, though it is of normal size. The sac around the testicle is filled with fluid making the testicle appear larger.

Trauma

Because of its location, the testicle is often traumatized. Sometimes it gets just a little bump. Other times, a misdirected football or baseball makes a man double up and see stars. Then there are the really unfortunate cases—coming down hard on a bike bar or a knee—that cause severe swelling. In our quest for preventive medicine, we strongly recommend wearing an athletic cup for all contact sports. Wear a jock strap (supporter) or briefs for all other, noncontact, sports. A jock strap holds the testicle closer to the body, making it a smaller target, and keeps the testicles from banging around.

A testicle that gets in the way of a baseball or knee or that is traumatized in any way will hurt. Because the nerves to the testicle come from the upper abdomen, you might feel pain in the stomach or back. If the scrotum or testicle swells, becomes black and blue, or continues to be painful, see a physician right away. The testicle may be torn, and some of its contents could spill out into the scrotum. This is called a ruptured testicle; it usually can be repaired surgically. If a rupture is not fixed right away, the testicle can shrink and stop producing sperm. So for those little hits that hurt, then go away, no big deal. But for the big hits that cause swelling, bruising, or persistent pain, see a doctor.

The Bottom Line

- The primary function of the testicles is to produce sperm and testosterone. Though men have a pair of testicles for this purpose, only one is usually needed. So, if one testicle has never been present or is lost from cryptorchidism, torsion, infection, or trauma, the remaining testicle is usually enough for adequate production of sperm and testosterone.

- All males, beginning at puberty, should do self-examinations of the testicles to make sure that there are no masses. Testicular cancer typically develops as a painless lump or bump, usually in young men. The treatment for testicular cancer is highly successful. Ignoring the mass or bump makes eventual treatment more difficult, and it can be fatal.

- Sudden onset of severe pain in the testicle is a medical emergency requiring prompt medical attention. Infection or torsion usually causes such pain. If the diagnosis is testicular torsion, or if the diagnosis is unknown, the male should go to the operating room for exploration and treatment.

- Long-term (chronic) scrotal pain is relatively common. All men will have some testicular pain at some point in their lives. If it persists, treatment should be sought. Some causes of testicular pain are varicoceles or infections. In most cases, clear causes are not found. In general, chronic scrotal pain should be treated conservatively.

- If the testicle is hit and there is swelling, bruising, or pain that does not go away, the male should see a physician as soon as possible. In most cases, everything will be fine. The physician will usually recommend treating the hurt scrotum/testicles with rest, ice, and pain medication. In the rare case of rupture, the testicle must be surgically repaired or it will be lost.

4

Premature Ejaculation
Stop, in the name of love

A recent article in the "medical" journal *Penthouse* (a magazine that sex doctors have to peruse to keep up on what's out there in the world of sex—really) says that 30 million American men suffer from premature ejaculation. This makes premature ejaculation the most common sexual problem among men.

What is premature ejaculation? Defining the problem is not easy. Masters and Johnson, pioneers in sex research, said a man has premature ejaculation if he cannot hold off long enough for the woman to have an orgasm 50 percent of the time. Well, how long does a guy have to last for most women to have an orgasm? In one study, 27 percent of women had orgasm when intercourse lasted less than a minute, whereas 66 percent had orgasm when intercourse lasted 12 minutes.

In the same study the average time for a women to have an orgasm was eight minutes. The problem with defining premature ejaculation as the inability of a man to hold off ejaculating long enough for a woman to have orgasm 50 percent of the time, is that orgasms vary so much from woman to woman. One woman may have an orgasm after a minute of sex every time. Others may never have one. If a woman never has an orgasm, does it mean her partner has premature ejaculation?

Others have tried to figure out how long intercourse typically takes and then define premature ejaculation as the length of time before ejaculation, regardless of whether the woman has an orgasm. Unfortunately, there is no consensus on how long intercourse lasts. In several surveys, the average length of intercourse was 20 minutes, in others about five minutes—quite a spread.

Still others have considered the number of thrusts. For example, if a man ejaculates with fewer than 15 thrusts, he has premature ejaculation. Surveys on this

32

subject, as you can well imagine, are hard to do. Most couples have a difficult time counting the number of thrusts during sex (and are they full thrusts, half-gainers, or what?). Finally, one manual claims a man has premature ejaculation if three criteria are fulfilled: The man ejaculates with minimal sexual stimulation before he wants to, it distresses the couple, and there is no substance abuse involved.

Virtually every male has premature ejaculation when he first experiences sex. One guy confided that when he was a teenager, he ejaculated after heavy kissing. This is just another example of learning how to have sex. If "spontaneous" ejaculation occurs, most guys just excuse themselves and go to the bathroom to clean up. With time, they develop some control over when they ejaculate. The same thing can occur when a man starts to have intercourse. There is so much excitement that it's over before you know it. Again, experience usually helps in developing control.

So ejaculating too quickly during the first few episodes is not premature ejaculation; it's normal. But after a man has some sexual experience under his belt, if ejaculation occurs too soon for him or his partner, it probably qualifies as premature ejaculation.

Then there are the men who have had no premature ejaculation in the past but suddenly develop it. What's going on there? Something new, such as an infection causing irritation or a problem with the relationship (also irritating) may have developed. But it's still premature ejaculation.

Evaluation and Treatment

The good news about premature ejaculation is that it is common. Anyone who has this problem need not feel singled out. The bad news is that it is often difficult to treat. In fact, it's probably worth trying some simple treatments at home before seeing a physician.

As mentioned above, a bit of time and experience may help a man relatively new to the joys of sex. If the problem persists, then some simple attempts to treat it are worthwhile. Condoms sometimes dull the sensation enough to delay ejaculation. If that doesn't work, try the *squeeze technique*, a good way to practice delaying ejaculation. With this technique, the man, or his partner, stimulates the penis. Right before he feels like he will ejaculate, one of them squeezes the head (glans) of the penis, which should inhibit ejaculation. Practice this several times before allowing ejaculation. The goal is to condition oneself not to ejaculate—it's penis training. The man can also focus on stimulating his partner while minimizing his own stimulation during foreplay so that they are more likely to climax together.

If a man has never suffered from this problem but suddenly finds himself coming too soon, he and his partner should take a look at what is new in their lives that might be causing this problem. In today's society there's plenty—from the plight of the world's hungry to the status of the pocketbook—to be stressed about. Stress can affect both a man and his relationship. Sleep, exercise, and—most important—talking and working things out with his partner may reduce stress, anxiety, and relationship problems. Dealing with these issues not only may help a man feel better about himself or help him and his partner feel better about their relationship, it also can help delay ejaculation.

If condoms, the squeeze, or stress-reducing techniques do not work, seek the help of a physician or sex therapist. If the problem seems to be physical, start with a urologist or a primary care physician. Expect the physician to do a thorough health history and physical examination to make sure there are no neurological problems (such as multiple sclerosis) or signs of infections (such as *prostatitis*). Both can cause premature ejaculation. Problems with erections should be discussed. A man with impotency may subconsciously ejaculate as soon as he can, before he loses the erection. Or anxiety about erections may cause him to ejaculate prematurely. Treat impotency first (see chapter 8); with successful treatment for impotency, premature ejaculation often goes away.

If a man thinks his premature ejaculation is likely the result of a psychological or couple problem, he should seek help from a sex therapist or a mental health counselor. Depression, anxiety, or relationship problems can cause premature ejaculation. These psychological issues may surface through simple questions or surveys. Depression often can be treated by medication; anxiety can be treated by medication or counseling; relationship issues are best dealt with in counseling.

Treatment is most effective when both a physician and a mental health counselor evaluate the situation and treat the patient together. But even with collaboration between health professionals, the specific cause for premature ejaculation may not be found. This makes premature ejaculation frustrating for everyone—the couple, physician, and counselor.

When no specific cause is evident, one of several medications may do the trick. Physicians have known for awhile that men taking antidepressants often complain about difficulties with ejaculation. In a moment of brilliancy, doctors realized that antidepressants might help men with premature ejaculation. We are not necessarily treating depression when we prescribe these drugs—we are just exploiting their known side effects.

For example, a couple recently came to our clinic complaining of premature ejaculation. They were both relatively new to sex. He had tried condoms to no avail. After finding nothing unusual in the physical examination and no obvious psychological or couple issues, we placed him on the antidepressant clomipramine. The good news about taking this medication for premature ejaculation is that he has to take it only before he wants to have sex. The bad thing is that he has to take it about 12 hours before he wants to have sex. Some of us can't figure out when we'll eat the next meal, much less when we'll be having sex. But our patient was able to plan ahead, and the medication worked. The treatment helped him "get over the hump," and now he does not need it. Others may need medication indefinitely for continued control of ejaculation.

Other medications such as Prozac® also are known to delay ejaculation. If one does not work, your physician may suggest another. But remember, these medications help because delaying ejaculation is a side effect. There can be other side effects such as a dry mouth or problems sleeping. But since the medications are taken in low doses or as a single dose before sex, these other side effects are rare.

Even if no cause is found, sex therapy, to learn new behaviors and techniques, and stress reduction may help a man gain control of ejaculation. Again, the best results seem to come from a combination of treatments, such as medication in conjunction with sex therapy.

As we learn more about the types and causes of premature ejaculation, the treatment options will improve. Undoubtedly, we'll see new medications specifically for the treatment of premature ejaculation. In the meantime, the man who is having problems with coming too soon should try one thing, then another, until he finds a therapy that works for him.

The Bottom Line

- Premature ejaculation is common among men of all ages.

- Ejaculating too soon often occurs when a guy is first experiencing sex. Unlike the characters in movies who act like they know what they're doing the first time, men and women in real life must learn sex. Until you have some experience, sex may produce anxiety that can cause premature ejaculation.

- Some men have no problems with premature ejaculation until later in their sexual lives. Something new, like a recent problem with erections or a new stress in a couple's life, may be the cause.

- Working to reduce stress, trying methods of relaxation, wearing condoms, and practicing the squeeze technique are easy ways to self-treat premature ejaculation.

- If home remedies don't work, see a sex therapist or a physician (a urologist or a primary care physician), according to whether you think the problem is physical or psychological. They will look for a specific cause and treat it.

- If no particular cause is found, any of several medications and behavior techniques may be helpful. Be persistent.

5

Male Infertility

Help sperm be all they can be

Right or wrong, the norm in most societies is for an individual to grow up, get a job, marry, and have children. So when couples are infertile, they carry a heavy emotional burden, both self-induced and from their support systems of family and friends. No wonder some couples are willing to mortgage their homes and spend thousands of dollars for the treatment of infertility.

Because of the stigma, couples who have difficulty conceiving a child often try to deal privately with their dilemma. This isolates them and makes them feel they have a rare problem. The reality is that infertility is a common problem. About 15 percent of all couples suffer from infertility.

Another misconception is that when a couple cannot conceive, the most likely cause is a problem with the female reproductive system. Clinical research shows that some infertile couples have a problem in the female, some in the male, and some in both. Overall if a couple is having problems conceiving, about 50 percent of the time the male has a problem with his sperm. This is not surprising. It takes both a man and a woman to make a baby. It's only fair the guy should be responsible for infertility half the time.

How do you know when you're infertile? The classic definition of infertility is one year of unprotected intercourse without conception. If the female partner has recently stopped taking birth-control pills and her periods are irregular, don't start counting until regular menstrual cycles have resumed. But if you suspect a problem with infertility because of an abnormal medical history, don't wait a year to seek evaluation. If a man has small testicles after having mumps as an adolescent, for instance, the couple might suspect some cause and effect and seek help right away. Other factors such as the age of the couple may affect fertility. If a couple is older, particularly if the woman is over age 35, they probably should seek help before a year passes.

Who should be evaluated? All too often one partner seeks evaluation and treatment before the other. This can waste time and money. Both partners should be evaluated simultaneously. One couple we know tried to conceive for a year before seeking help. The woman was evaluated and placed on *clomiphene citrate* (a drug used to regulate the cycle and increase the number of eggs) for a year. Eventually, a semen analysis was obtained which showed that the man had no sperm. This woman was inappropriately treated with a costly medication that can have unpleasant side effects. Since the husband had no sperm, the treatment was a waste of time as well. If only he had been checked out at the very beginning!

Women often seek evaluation for infertility long before their male partners. For efficient, timely, and cost-effective results, however, both partners should be assessed simultaneously. Male assessment must go beyond a semen analysis, as semen does not tell the whole story. For example, sperm may be present and moving okay, but unable to bind or fertilize the egg. A good health history and physical examination can point out potential problems with sperm function. Identifying the problem is the first step to treatment. A health history, physical examination, and semen analysis are all part of a thorough evaluation for male infertility.

Anatomy: Sizing Up Testicles

We touched on the anatomy of the scrotum and its contents (the testicle, epididymis, and vas deferens) earlier, but more must be said about the size of testicles. Remember that a testicle is made up primarily of sperm. So if a testicle is small, it may not be making much sperm.

What is considered small? A testicle that is less than an inch-and-a-half from top to bottom is small. But we warn you—it's tough to measure the testicle. It doesn't count to measure the scrotum, just the testicle itself. A lot of skin and fluid can get in the way of gauging testicular size. If a man has a hydrocele, for example, he may appear to have a big testicle. But because of all the fluid in the hydrocele, he may not even be able to feel his testicle, much less measure it.

A small testicle is sometimes called an *atrophic testicle*. This can occur for many reasons. An undescended (cryptorchid) testicle, even after being brought down into the scrotum by orchiopexy, may be small. Trauma, torsion, infection, and the presence of a varicocele are among the many other reasons a testicle may be atrophic. A genetic or hormonal problem also can affect the size, usually of both testicles.

Remember, a man needs just one good testicle to conceive. Considering how important the preservation of the species is from an evolutionary standpoint and where the testicles are located, it's nice to have a spare! So one small testicle may not cause a man to be infertile. To further complicate matters, there are many exceptions to the size of the testicle correlating to sperm production. Some men with small testicles produce lots of sperm, whereas some with big testicles produce little or none. Reproduction is complex.

Evaluation of the Patient with Male Infertility

An infertility evaluation need not be done by a specialist. But since reproduction is complicated, you will want someone who is knowledgeable and who has an interest in fertility and reproduction. For women, this usually means an obstetrician/gynecologist or a *reproductive endocrinologist*. For men, a urologist with a strong interest in reproduction fits the bill. In some cases, a primary-care physician familiar with infertility does the initial evaluation. If the process becomes complicated, if a difficult problem is encountered, or if things take too long, the infertile couple may wish to see an infertility specialist.

Since there are hundreds of potential causes for male infertility, a detailed medical history is important. The doctor should ask whether the man has had developmental problems or childhood illnesses. For example, undescended testicles (cyptorchidism), surgery on the bladder, mumps as a teenager, or delayed puberty could affect fertility.

A history of current illnesses, such as diabetes, is important. So is a list of current medications. Some medications, such as sulfasalazine for ulcerative colitis, cimetidine for gastritis and peptic ulcer disease, and nitrofurantoin for urinary tract infections, can harm the testicles and sperm. Some medications cause problems with ejaculation. Smoking, excess alcohol consumption, and recreational drugs, including marijuana, also hurt the testicles. Steroids may help a guy get big muscles, but they won't make his testicles larger. In fact, steroids shrink testicles and harm sperm production.

Exposure to chemotherapy, radiation therapy, solvents, paints, pesticides, and heat (frequent use of saunas or hot tubs), can also harm a man's testicles and affect the production of sperm. The patient's assessment of stress factors is also important. The doctor should ask about the man's sexual history, including problems with ejaculation or erections. These sexual problems inevitably lead to a decreased frequency of intercourse. It's hard to get pregnant if you don't have sex!

Finally, the physician will want a general history of other organs, such as lungs, heart, and nervous system. Difficulty with vision may seem to have little to do with fertility, but an abnormal pituitary gland can cause problems with peripheral vision and sperm production. Hundreds of questions may be needed to pinpoint the cause of infertility. Most require short answers. But complete information is important to determine appropriate treatment.

Next is the physical examination, usually focused on the penis, testicles, and prostate gland. The most important part of the examination is to check out the scrotum and its contents. The physician checks the testicles inside the scrotum to make sure they are of normal size and consistency. As mentioned earlier, if a testicle is small or very soft, it probably does not produce sperm well. The physician also feels carefully for a varicocele (dilated veins that feel like a bag of worms). The epididymis and vas deferens are also examined to make sure that they are present and feel normal. Finally, though never popular, a rectal examination assures that the prostate is of the right size and consistency and is not tender. Tenderness can be a sign of a prostate infection that contributes to infertility.

Laboratory Testing

Semen is the fluid that is ejaculated; it normally contains sperm. A good semen analysis is critical for evaluating infertility. When a laboratory looks at semen, it checks the volume (amount) of ejaculate and the concentration (count) of sperm. It also checks the *motility* (how many sperm are moving) and shape of sperm (called *morphology*). Typically, we like to see at least two milliliters (mls) of ejaculate (half-a-teaspoonful), at least 20 million sperm per ml for the sperm concentration, at least 50 percent of the sperm moving, and a least 30 percent of the sperm with normal shape. Other factors such as white blood cells and how many sperm are living are sometimes measured as well.

In a normal individual, sperm concentration can vary tremendously and change more than the Dow Jones Industrial Average. It is not unusual for sperm count to vary from none to hundreds of millions per ml. So at least two, and sometimes three, semen samples are needed to see whether a man has a problem with sperm production.

In addition, the morphology or shape of the sperm gives some idea of its functioning. Having abnormally shaped sperm does not necessarily mean there are DNA or genetic problems. It may mean simply that the sperm does not function well. The traditional criteria is for 30 percent of sperm to be of normal shape. There is another criteria, called the *Krueger's strict criteria*, for analyzing sperm shape. Using this method, abnormal is defined as having less than 15 percent of sperm normal in shape. In other words, having up to 85 percent abnormal-shaped sperm is normal. Higher rates of abnormal sperm may indicate a problem with sperm function.

To minimize fluctuation in sperm count, motility, and morphology, samples must be collected in a standard fashion. We encourage patients to abstain from sex two to five days before collecting a sample. This may vary slightly from lab to lab, but it is a good overall standard.

Semen samples are collected by masturbation into a sterile container. The clinic will provide a special container, since others may have substances that can hurt sperm or affect the semen analysis. Men have been known to bring samples in Tupperware®, ketchup bottles, mayonnaise jars, baby-food jars, with and without ribbons attached. We don't want to limit your imagination, but the sterile container provided by the lab will give the most accurate results.

Collecting samples at the clinic also gives better results. The clinic should provide a private, secure, and quiet room for collecting the sample. This way the sample can be analyzed shortly after it is collected. With too much delay between collection and analysis, the sperm may die or show abnormal values.

Normal Sperm

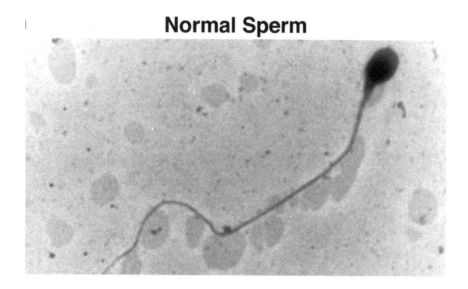

Abnormal Sperm

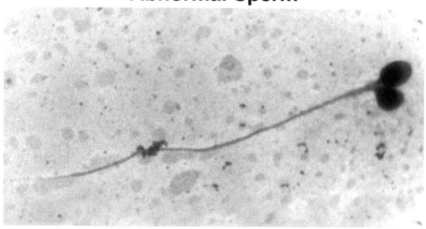

At top, normal-shaped sperm. At bottom, abnormal-shaped (two-headed) sperm.

In addition to analyzing sperm, some laboratories look for round cells. Round cells may look like white blood cells and lead to a misdiagnosis of infection. Sometimes the cells truly are white blood cells, and the patient indeed has an infection. But in most cases, the round cells are immature sperm that have not elongated and so do not look typical. Too many immature sperm means a problem with sperm production. In such cases, treatment with antibiotics is inappropriate. So you will want to know whether the laboratory can distinguish white blood cells from immature sperm. Usually the lab must stain the specimen to distinguish between the two.

All men have some white blood cells in their semen. This is normal. But too many white blood cells, usually more than a million per milliliter, may indicate an infection. If the doctor says there is a prostate infection based on a semen analysis, ask whether the lab can distinguish white blood cells from immature sperm. Ask, too, how many white blood cells there are and for a culture to verify infection.

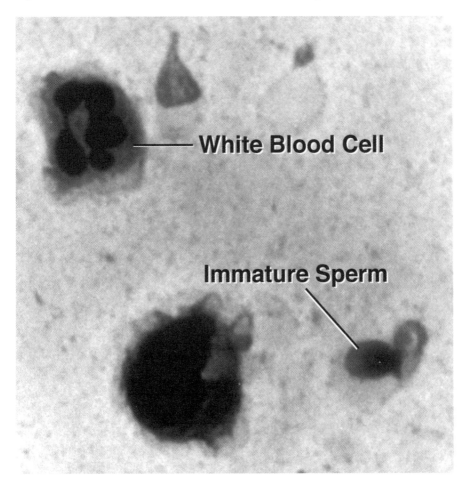

The white blood cell at left appears identical to the immature, round sperm cell at right. It's easy to see why immature sperm are often mistaken for white blood cells—and the man told he has an infection of the prostate.

All men being evaluated for infertility should have a history, physical examination, and at least two semen analyses. Depending on the results of these, additional testing may be necessary to determine whether there is a fertility problem and why. Such testing commonly includes drawing some blood for a check of hormone levels— testosterone, *follicle stimulating hormone (FSH)*, and *prolactin*. Hormones may affect testicles. The health of testicles in turn affects hormone levels in the bloodstream.

Other tests, such as checking for *antisperm antibodies*, are sometimes helpful. This test determines whether a man's antibodies are attacking his own sperm. It can also screen for antibodies in a woman's blood or cervical mucus that might be attacking her partner's sperm.

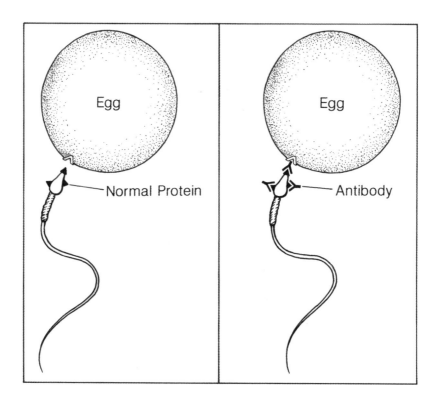

At left, the triangles on the sperm represent proteins necessary for the sperm to bind to the egg. At right, antibodies attacking the proteins keep the sperm from binding to the egg making the man infertile.

The hamster test (also called the sperm penetration assay or SPA) is another analysis that is sometimes done. With this test, a sperm sample is mixed with the eggs of a hamster to get some idea of how well the sperm functions and fertilizes eggs. The covering of the hamster eggs, which can be penetrated only by hamster sperm, is removed to allow healthy human sperm to penetrate the eggs. Of course, we do not have hamster people. Once human sperm penetrates the hamster egg, the process stops because of the biochemical and genetic differences between hamsters and humans.

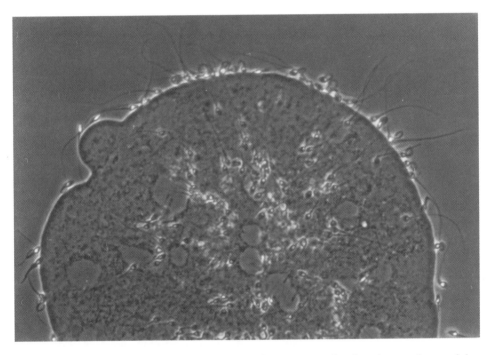

In the hamster test, or sperm penetration assay, human sperm bind to the egg. Some of the sperm have penetrated the egg, which indicates good sperm function.

On occasion, *transrectal ultrasound (TRUS)* is used to look at a man's reproductive system. TRUS uses sound waves instead of x-rays, which are harmful to sperm. It's not as bad as it sounds. A probe is inserted into the rectum to identify blockage in the prostate that might be preventing the full ejaculate from coming out. Scrotal ultrasound is sometimes used to screen for varicoceles, measure for testicular size, and look for signs of infection or blockage.

Causes and Treatment of Infertility

There are hundreds and hundreds of potential causes for infertility in men. Often, a man's infertility has more than one cause. Some are easily identified, but others are not. Likewise, some are correctable, others not.

A varicocele (dilated vein in the scrotum) is the most common correctable problem. We do not know exactly how varicoceles cause infertility. Most specialists believe they disrupt the cooling mechanism of the testes, causing the testicles to overheat. This in turn decreases sperm production or interferes with sperm function. As discussed in chapter 3, varicoceles may be treated by surgery (varicocelectomy) or by radiology (embolization). Complete recovery from the radiology procedure is faster (1–2 days). But the surgical approach is usually preferred because of its lower risks and costs.

As mentioned, antisperm antibodies can cause infertility. Sperm is like a foreign cell to the rest of a man's body. This occurs because the sperm take on many new proteins during maturation (at puberty) that the immune system has not seen before. Sperm is to a man as pollen is to someone with hay fever. The sperm hide from the immune system in the testicle, where a barrier keeps blood and white blood cells away from them. This prevents a man's allergic reaction to his own sperm. Sometimes, however, the immune system does see sperm and makes antibodies to attack them. These antisperm antibodies (ASA) may affect sperm motility or function, or cause sperm clumping.

At present we are unable to remove antibodies from sperm without damaging the sperm. One possible treatment is steroids for the man and simultaneous intrauterine insemination for the couple (putting sperm directly into the uterus, discussed later in this chapter). Steroids may have some serious side effects. Be sure to discuss the potential side effects with a physician before embarking on steroid therapy. If this treatment fails to reduce the antibodies or result in a pregnancy, in vitro fertilization (also discussed later in this chapter) is commonly recommended.

An infection in any reproductive organ, from testicle to prostate, can injure or cause clumping of the sperm. Severe infections can scar or block the tubes that carry sperm. Treatment begins after testing the semen to determine what type of bacteria is present and what type of antibiotics will work the best. Routinely a week or so of antibiotics kill the bacteria. Usually both partners are treated simultaneously.

Since hormones are necessary for the production and maintenance of sperm, hormonal problems can cause infertility. The pituitary gland, in the middle of the brain, secretes follicle-stimulating hormone (FSH) and *luteinizing hormone (LH)*, which react with the testicle. FSH stimulates *Sertoli cells* in the testicle, which support and nurture sperm. LH stimulates cells that make testosterone, which is necessary for sperm production. Naturally, problems with LH, FSH, and other hormones can affect fertility. But these substances are easily measured in blood, and imbalances are treatable.

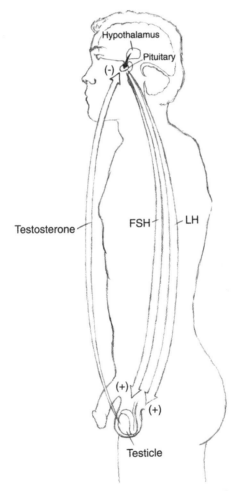

The hypothalamus controls the pituitary gland. (Both are in the brain.) The pituitary gland secretes FSH and LH into the blood and stimulates the testicles. The testicles, in turn, make substances, such as testosterone, that get into the bloodstream and tell the pituitary and hypothalamus to slow down—"don't make so much FSH and LH." In this way the hypothalamus, pituitary gland, and testicle "talk" to each other.

The treatment, of course, depends on which hormone is abnormal. Several medications are available to return the semen to normal limits or at least improve its quality.

Obstruction or a blockage can cause infertility. Remember, sperm are made in the testicle. Then they go through a highly coiled tube called the epididymis, which is located behind the testicle, then through the vas deferens. The vas deferens goes behind the bladder and through the prostate, where the sperm mix with fluid from the prostate and seminal vesicle as they are ejaculated. A blockage of the epididymis, the vas deferens, or around the prostate can decrease the number and motility of sperm.

Obstruction at the epididymis can be congenital (developed before birth). Or it may be caused by infection, trauma, or vasectomy (*epididymal blowout,* see chapter 7, on vasectomy reversal). Blockages or obstructions of the vas deferens most commonly are caused by vasectomy or other previous surgery such as hernia repair. Prostate or seminal vesicle obstruction may be congenital or caused by infection. In some cases, obstruction is so severe that no sperm at all are evident. This is called *azoospermia—* no sperm.

In many cases obstructions are treatable. If a man has no sperm (is azoospermic), he should have a *retrograde semen analysis* to determine whether there is sperm in the urine. In case of little or no sperm in the retrograde sample, a TRUS will determine whether the blockage lies in the prostate. If the ultrasound proves normal, the next step is surgical biopsy of the testicle. This small procedure (it takes 10–15 minutes) determines whether the testicle produces sperm normally. A normal biopsy implies a blockage, usually at the epididymis or vas deferens if the prostate was shown to be normal by the TRUS. An abnormal biopsy implies no blockage; the testicle apparently does not make enough sperm to show in the ejaculate.

Anyone undergoing testicular biopsy should not have a *vasogram* (an x-ray that looks for blockage of the vas deferens) at the same time. Though the dose of radiation from the vasogram is too low to hurt the testicle, the needle used to inject contrast into the vas deferens can injure the vas deferens. A vasogram should be done only when the blockage is being repaired, which is usually not at the time of the biopsy. Once a blockage is confirmed, repair may be performed. The surgery needed depends on the location of the obstruction.

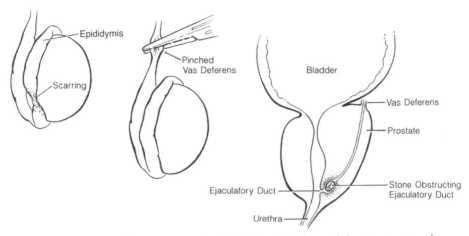

Three common areas where sperm can be blocked: at left the epididymis, at center the vas deferens, and at right the ejaculatory duct. The epididymis is the most common place for blockage.

Poisons, x-rays, and things harmful to the testicle are called gonadotoxins. Many substances—in the environment, in the food we eat, in the medicines we take, and in the activities we pursue—affect sperm production. For example, heat kills sperm (watch out for those hot tubs). Wearing boxer shorts so the testicles can "hang in the breeze" probably doesn't help fertility much. But wearing boxers can't hurt, so go ahead and enjoy them.

Smoking, drinking alcohol excessively, and exposure to certain chemicals such as pesticides, insecticides, or fumes from a factory can affect sperm. A man who has undergone chemotherapy or radiation therapy for cancer may have a fertility problem (these therapies kill sperm as well as cancer). Some of these substances cannot be avoided; with others we should try. It takes three months for sperm to mature, so we must wait three months or longer to find out whether removing a substance has a positive effect on sperm production. In some cases the semen analysis returns to normal with time. In others the damage is permanent.

In recent years, exploring genetic causes for infertility has been a hot topic. Many researchers, including this author, have pursued it. Most of the genes responsible for testicular development and sperm production are located on the Y *chromosome* (referred to by some as the male chromosome). Recent studies show a link between missing parts of the Y chromosome and infertility. We can now test men to find out whether they are missing part of their Y chromosome.

Men who have cystic fibrosis or are carriers of the cystic fibrosis gene also may have a genetic cause for infertility. The gene that causes cystic fibrosis can hinder development of the vas deferens. In men without a vas deferens, sperm can't leave the testicle.

Many other genetic problems may cause infertility. Treatment depends on the specific disorder. For example, if a guy is missing his vas deferens on both sides, sperm may be retrieved from the testicle by testicular sperm extraction (TESE). Then in vitro fertilization with sperm injection (intracytoplasmic sperm injection or ICSI) can be done (see next section, on assisted reproduction technologies). In cases for which no treatment is known, most patients are consoled by finally having an answer as to why they are unable to conceive.

Another treatable cause of infertility is a problem with ejaculation. Difficulty with ejaculation can occur because of a spinal cord injury, diabetes, or previous surgery. A man may have *retrograde ejaculation* (semen going back into the bladder instead of out the end of the penis) or *anejaculation* (orgasm with no semen or fluid going out the penis). Ejaculation may be induced in these cases. A medication may produce an ejaculate or bring the semen from the bladder out the end of the penis. In the case of spinal cord injury, a vibrator placed on a specific area on the penis or a probe placed in the rectum that releases tiny electrical impulses can cause ejaculation. The specimen is collected, then inserted into the woman's uterus during ovulation. These procedures, done in fertility clinics, must be carefully timed.

Finally, some men have *idiopathic infertility*. This means we cannot exactly identify the problem. Sometimes medications like clomiphene citrate improve sperm counts in men with idiopathic infertility. Other medications may improve sperm motility. For example, a dietary supplement called Proxeed® has been shown in some studies to improve sperm movement. The primary ingredient in Proxeed® is carnitine, which is like an amino acid and is found in some foods. Proxeed® must be taken twice a day for at least six months before a physician can know whether sperm movement has improved. You can find information on this supplement, which does not require a prescription, on the Internet (see Appendix 2).

Clomiphene citrate, Proxeed®, and other medications or dietary supplements that can improve sperm production are a kind of *empirical therapy*—treatment that has a theoretical basis for working but has not yet been proven. Empirical therapy is fine, but any guy who tries it upon a physician's advice should be aware that no cause for his infertility has been found. There should be follow-up. At the end of six months, the patient should know whether the medication is working. If not, the therapy should end so that the couple can move on to other options (see below).

Assisted Reproductive Technologies

When the cause of infertility is unknown or the treatments discussed earlier do not result in a pregnancy, couples may choose to advance to assisted reproductive technology (ART). Intrauterine insemination is one of these treatments. With intrauterine insemination, a gynecologist with a background in female infertility inserts the male partner's sperm into the female's uterus at the time of ovulation.

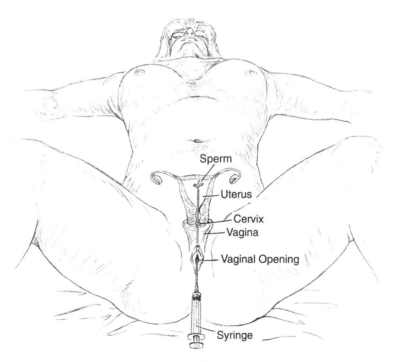

Sperm are injected into the uterus during intrauterine insemination.

In-vitro fertilization (IVF) is more complex. Basically it results in a "test-tube baby." With IVF, the woman takes hormones to increase the number of eggs she produces each month. At the time of ovulation, the eggs are removed from her ovaries. The male produces a semen sample through masturbation or, in cases of no sperm in the ejaculate, a surgeon removes the sperm from the testicle (testicular sperm extraction or TESE). The sperm and the eggs meet in a petri dish, and we wait for fertilization to occur. Sometimes the sperm must be injected into the eggs in a procedure called intracytoplasmic sperm injection (ICSI). If IVF is necessary and there is male infertility, ICSI is the best way to help the sperm fertilize the eggs. Once fertilized, the eggs are reimplanted in the woman's uterus. IVF is expensive and success rates vary tremendously from clinic to clinic. Research the clinics you are interested in for the best chance of success.

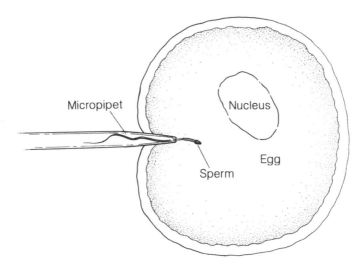

Sperm is injected directly into the egg with intracytoplasmic sperm injection (ICSI). This is a great technique when there is no other treatment for an infertile male, especially one with very low sperm counts. For men with no sperm in their ejaculate, sperm often can be extracted from the testicle (testicular sperm extraction, TESE) and used for ICSI.

Donor Insemination and Adoption

There are alternatives to using a mate's sperm to conceive. Donor insemination can be less expensive than other options. Most sperm banks require donors to meet strict qualifications and undergo extensive disease prescreening before participating in their programs. Couples may review donor catalogs giving brief descriptions of a donor's looks, social and family background, and some medical information. Once a donor is chosen, the sample is thawed and inseminated into the female partner at the time of ovulation. This procedure takes place at a fertility clinic. The wonderful part of using a donor is that you get to enjoy the pregnancy and birth of your child.

Adoption is an alternative to using the man's sperm or assisted reproductive techniques. Nowadays many different organizations are available to help arrange many different kinds of adoptions. Support groups for infertility, such as Resolve, can provide lists of adoption agencies and organizations. Just look in your phone book to find a local group.

The Bottom Line

- Whatever the reason for a couple's infertility, both partners should be evaluated by a physician knowledgeable about infertility.

- There are hundreds of potential causes for male infertility, and more than one problem may be identified. Some problems are easily identified and corrected; others are not.

- A medical history, physical examination, and at least two semen analyses should be part of every evaluation for male infertility. Additional testing may be necessary to determine whether a man has a fertility problem and why.

- The development of assisted reproductive technologies (ART) has helped more and more couples to conceive. But couples should be prepared to pay a steep financial and emotional price.

- Usually persistence, medical treatment, and a bit of luck will result in a pregnancy. If a couple cannot have a child "biologically," donor insemination and adoption are other great ways to start a family.

6

Vasectomy
Snip-snip

Excruciating pain, being bedridden for weeks, impotency, and worst of all, no ejaculation during intercourse—these are some of the ideas (and excuses) men think of when they consider a vasectomy. Recent reports of vasectomy associated with prostate cancer have not helped to allay their fears. The truth is, a vasectomy is a relatively easy procedure usually followed by an uneventful course, and it is a reliable form of birth control.

Anatomy and Function of the Vas Deferens

Sperm are made in the testicle. They make their way through the *epididymis*, located behind the testicle. The epididymis is a single, very thin, highly coiled tube that begins at the top of the testis and works its way toward the bottom. Sperm mature and become capable of fertilizing as they travel through this tube. They are stored in the bottom, or tail, of the epididymis. During ejaculation, sperm leave the epididymis and go through a tube called the vas *deferens*.

The vas deferens is a thick-walled tube about the size of a spaghetti noodle but much firmer. You can feel the vas deferens in the scrotum as it courses from the tail of the epididymis towards the inguinal canal, an area located at the top of the thigh. The vas deferens then travels down into the pelvis and behind the bladder as it goes through the prostate gland into the urethra. The vas deferens carries sperm and a small amount of fluid from the testicle and epididymis to the urethra and out the end of the penis.

Sperm cells make up only 1 percent of ejaculate. Most of the fluid that comes out during ejaculation is from the seminal vesicles. These winglike structures near the prostate contribute fluid and substances that help sperm move and escape detection

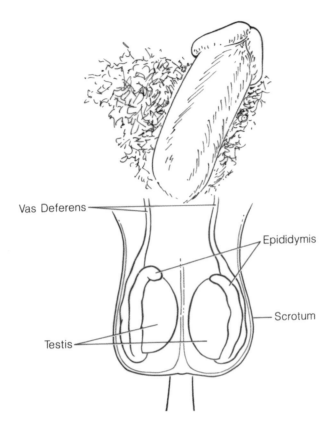

Sperm are made in the testicle and stored in the epididymis. Ejaculation propels the sperm through the vas deferens on its way to the prostate and beyond. The vas deferens is tied off on both sides for a vasectomy.

from the female's immune system. A significant amount of fluid also comes from the prostate gland, which helps maintain the life of the sperm. So when the vas deferens is cut in a vasectomy, there should be no detectable change in the amount, color, or consistency of the fluid (semen) that comes from ejaculation. The only change is a lack of sperm.

Who Gets and Who Should Get a Vasectomy

About 500,000 men get vasectomies in the United States each year. Virtually any adult male of any age can get one. Many physicians want patients considering a vasectomy to be married and to have several children, but these are not medical requirements.

Although a vasectomy can be reversed, reversal is not always successful and it can be expensive. So consider a vasectomy a permanent form of birth control. Ask yourself whether you would want more children if you separated from your partner, if your partner died, or if one of your children died. If you do not want more children under any circumstances, a vasectomy is a good choice for birth control.

A man can bank (i.e. freeze) his sperm before a vasectomy is performed. But it is expensive, and most men, convinced at the time of vasectomy that they want no more children, decide against it.

The Procedure

A urologist or family practitioner (or sometimes a general surgeon) typically performs vasectomies as an outpatient procedure at a hospital or clinic. In other words, the patient goes home the same day. The cost varies, usually between $250 and $500. Typically a vasectomy is covered by insurance (it's cheaper than having a baby). Check your specific coverage to be sure. Before a vasectomy, the patient will be asked to sign a consent form stating that he understands the risks and that a vasectomy is considered permanent.

For the procedure, the hair is shaved from the scrotum to make the vasectomy go more easily and quickly. Most of the pubic hair is left in place. The area is scrubbed with a prepping solution (one hopes a warm prepping solution) to kill all the bacteria. The physician then holds the vas deferens between his/her fingers and injects a local anesthetic to numb the area. Usually this is the only part of the procedure that hurts. Using a very small needle minimizes the sting.

Next, a small incision, about half-an-inch long, is made in the scrotum, and the vas deferens is grasped. A piece of the vas deferens is then cut off. This piece of tissue often is sent to a pathologist to make sure it is from the vas deferens. The physician then clips or ties the vas deferens to block the two ends from which the segment was removed. Some surgeons also burn one or both ends with an electric cautery instrument. This causes the tissue to scar and prevents sperm from the testicular end of the vas deferens from finding its way to the abdominal end of the vas deferens. Finally, many physicians suture the ends of the vas deferens at different levels so that they can't grow back together. The incision is then closed with one or two absorbable sutures. After one side is done, the physician repeats the vasectomy on the other side. The whole procedure usually takes 10–30 minutes (5–15 minutes per side) depending on the skill of the physician and the ease of locating and holding the vas deferens.

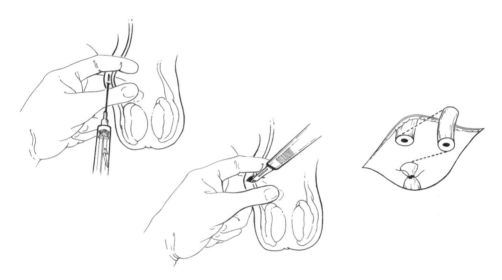

A tiny needle is used to numb the scrotum and vas deferens. A small incision is made over the vas deferens and a small segment of the vas cut out. Often, one end of the vas is burned and the other tied off. The same procedure is done on the opposite vas. The entire procedure is pain-free (except for the numbing) and takes about 20 minutes.

The No-Scalpel Vasectomy

A vasectomy also can be performed without an incision. This is called the *no-scalpel vasectomy* technique. Instead of an incision, the surgeon grabs the vas deferens with a special clamp that brings it closer to the skin and punctures a small hole in the skin around the vas deferens with another clamp. The vas deferens is pulled up through the puncture hole. The rest of the vasectomy is performed as described above (cutting out a segment of the vas and tying or burning the ends). The advantage of this technique is that in experienced hands it is quicker and can result in less postoperative pain. The disadvantage is that pulling the vas deferens through a puncture is more difficult than pulling it through an incision. The no-scalpel vasectomy requires greater surgical experience.

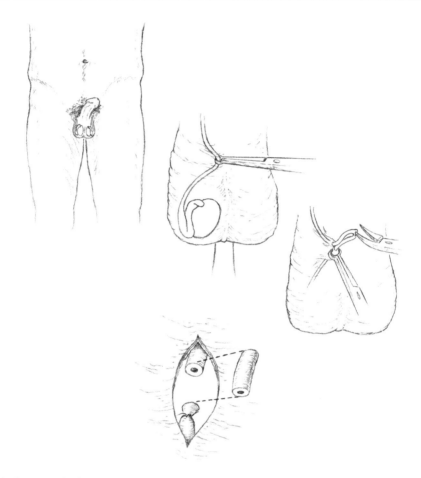

With the no-scalpel vasectomy technique, a puncture is made in the middle of the scrotum. A special clamp grasps one vas and pulls it out. The vasectomy is then completed as with the traditional technique. After one side is done, the other vas is brought out through the same puncture hole. This is a useful but somewhat-tricky technique.

Care after a Vasectomy

The patient should bring a jock strap to the doctor's office at the time of the vasectomy because it will give support and comfort during the following week. It's not a good idea to play football, hockey, or have intercourse right after a vasectomy. In fact, you may not want to do anything strenuous for the first week. Wait a week before intercourse or masturbation. The vasectomy site must heal before it is subjected to strenuous activity.

Remember that after the vas deferens is tied off, some sperm remains in both ends of the vas deferens. Intercourse can still result in a pregnancy. So continue to use birth control until the physician tells you that no sperm is left in the ejaculate. Typically it takes two to four months for the system to "clean out." To be sure the system is clear, ejaculate about 20 times over a ten-week period, then bring a semen sample to the physician's office or clinic to be examined for sperm. Do this twice. In other words, before having intercourse without protection, you need two semen analyses to show that no sperm remains in the ejaculate.

Risk and Problems with Vasectomies

Most vasectomies are performed without complications. Occasionally some bruising, pain, or slight bleeding occurs. This usually goes away on its own. If a man has continued bleeding, he should put pressure on the scrotum at the incision site and call his physician if it does not stop. Occasionally, severe bleeding occurs and the scrotum swells, sometimes larger than a softball. If this happens, the patient should be seen immediately, by the physician who did the vasectomy if possible. In about 3 percent of patients, infection occurs. Drainage of yellowish fluid, pain, redness, and heat around the area of the incision are signs of an infection. If there are signs of an infection, antibiotics and local wound treatment may be needed.

There's a one-in-a-thousand chance that the two ends of the vas deferens will eventually find each other and form a new track for sperm to get from the testicle to the urethra. This is called *recanalization*. In other words, even though a vasectomy is supposed to be permanent, the procedure does not always work. The only absolutely sure method of birth control for a man is abstinence or removal of the testicles. Most guys find neither of these attractive and so accept the one-in-a-thousand chance of recanalization and possible pregnancy, which are better odds than most other forms of birth control.

Some recent reports have suggested a connection between prostate cancer and vasectomy. Follow-up studies show that prostate cancer does not occur more often in men who have vasectomies. One explanation for the discrepancies among studies may be that men who undergo vasectomy are more health-conscious. Since men who have had vasectomies tend to see physicians more often, prostate cancer is detected more frequently in this group. Prostate cancer is not more likely to occur, it is just more likely to be found, in men who see their physicians. There is no known biological reason that prostate cancer would occur more often in men with vasectomies. So while the studies continue, we believe it safe to say a vasectomy does not increase your chances of getting prostate cancer.

Finally, scrotal pain, referred to as post-vasectomy pain syndrome, occurs in a small percentage of patients. Apparently, because the vas deferens is blocked, sperm building up in the epididymis causes it to swell. The increased pressure in the epididymis causes pain in the rare patient with this problem. Usually hot baths, aspirin, and time take care of it, but on occasion more invasive treatment is needed. One remedy is removal of the epididymis. Another is to reconnect the vas deferens in a procedure called vasovasostomy (see chapter 7). The down side to a vasovasostomy is that with reversal, some new form of birth control will be needed. Most men have some scrotal pain after a vasectomy; occasional pain around the testicles is usually nothing to worry about. But if the pain is persistent, see your physician.

The Bottom Line

- Vasectomies are common and relatively easy to perform. They are easier to do and result in fewer complications than tubal ligations for women. It seems fair to us that if the woman carries and delivers the children, the least that the man can do is undergo a vasectomy when the time comes to stop having them.

- Before getting a vasectomy, carefully consider the consequences of the procedure. Think of this as a permanent form of birth control.

- A man undergoing a vasectomy should use another form of birth control until his physician tells him, after two separate tests, that no sperm remains in the semen.

7

Vasectomy Reversal
Change your mind?

As we have said, you should consider a vasectomy to be permanent. So why are we discussing vasectomy reversals? Well, a vasectomy is reversible; it's just that the reversal is not always successful. Besides, everyone knows life is full of the unexpected. Changes such as divorce and remarriage or the loss of a loved one can create a desire for more children.

For whatever reasons, people do change their minds, and they are free to do so at any time after a vasectomy. One man called to ask how much a reversal would cost. That in itself was not unusual, but the fact that he called two hours after his vasectomy was. Others call many years later. It is not unusual for men to have a vasectomy reversed as many as 15 to 20 years later.

Vasovasostomy

A *vasovasostomy* is a reconnection of the vas deferens. Under most circumstances, the two ends of vas deferens cut during a vasectomy can be reattached. This is referred to as *anastomosis* of the vas. It is done as an outpatient procedure.

The best way to do a vasovasostomy is under a microscope using microsurgical techniques. Microsurgery is a specialized skill that requires continued practice to maintain a high level of expertise. A surgeon who performs at least 25 vasectomy reversals a year should have the expertise you want. A microsurgical vasovasostomy is usually performed by a urologist, though some plastic surgeons also do it.

For a vasovasostomy, the patient goes to sleep or is under local anesthesia. The scrotum is shaved and prepped with a special solution to kill all the bacteria. A small incision is made in the scrotum, and the two previously cut ends of the vas deferens are found. One end comes from the testicle; the other leads to the urethra. The surgeon cuts a small segment from each to freshen the ends and make sure they are open. Then, under the microscope, the surgeon reattaches the vas with sutures smaller than a hair. The vas deferens on both left and right sides is reconnected. The entire procedure takes two to three hours.

A dressing (bandage) and jock strap are placed on the scrotum. The patient recovers in the recovery room and goes home later that day. Heavy lifting, intercourse, and masturbation must be avoided for four weeks. Several months after the operation, a semen analysis is obtained to determine its success. Frequently, the first semen analysis will show a low sperm count and/or low motility (sperm movement). This usually gets better with time. Intercourse should be timed to when the woman ovulates.

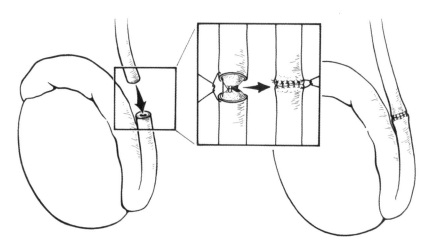

In a vasovasostomy, both ends of the vas are reconnected under a microscope with sutures smaller than a hair.

The success rate of vasovasostomy is good. Ninety to 95 percent of cases show sperm in the ejaculate (in other words, the vas is open or patent) and 50 to 70 percent of couples have a pregnancy. The reason the pregnancy rate is not higher is that there can be other fertility problems present in one partner or the other. Remember, 15 percent of all couples are infertile to begin with. Also, a vasectomy can cause permanent damage to the testicle or the epididymis.

One example of such damage is the formation of antisperm antibodies experienced by a majority of the patients who have had a vasectomy. Antibodies are molecules made by the immune system to attack foreign material. As discussed earlier, a man's immune system views sperm, which in a sense is hidden in the testicle, as foreign. After a vasectomy, sperm is still produced; it is absorbed by the epididymis. This absorption exposes sperm to the immune system, which may produce antibodies. These antibodies sometimes attach themselves to the sperm and prevent the sperm from functioning by lowering their motility or preventing them from binding to eggs. Usually antisperm antibodies go away after a reversal, so you don't need to check for them beforehand. But if there is no pregnancy a year after reversal, you should check for antisperm antibodies as well as other causes of infertility.

On average, pregnancy occurs about one year after a vasectomy reversal. Remember what *average* means. One man who underwent vasectomy seven years ago came into our clinic wanting his vasectomy reversed. He was getting married in six months. We explained that on average it takes about a year after reversal for pregnancy to occur. The couple thought this would be perfect as the wedding was half a year away. A vasectomy reversal (vasovasostomy) was performed without difficulty. A month later we told him he could resume all normal activity. The first time the couple had intercourse, she got pregnant. The two were not yet married, but they had a good sense of humor and were pleased that the procedure had worked. A pregnancy can occur at any time, but in some cases it does not happen at all.

The Treatment for Epididymal Blowout

An epididymal blowout can occur sometime after a vasectomy. Remember, after a vasectomy the sperm have nowhere to go because the end of the vas is tied off. The testicle keeps on making sperm, which keep going through the epididymis until they run into the obstruction. The epididymis becomes more and more filled with sperm. White blood cells in the epididymis digest the sperm, but sometimes there are just too many to keep up with. Eventually the small, fragile epididymal tubule may rupture. This is epididymal blowout. Scar tissue forms at the site of rupture, creating a block in the epididymal tubule. Since there is only one epididymal tubule carrying sperm from the testicle to the vas deferens, there is a blockage not only at the site of the vasectomy but also the epididymis. So if a vasovasostomy is performed at the site of the previous vasectomy and there is blockage in the epididymis, the sperm cannot make its way into the ejaculate.

The longer the time since vasectomy, the more likely epididymal blowout will occur. At ten years after vasectomy about 50 percent of patients have had epididymal blowout. Though epididymal blowout sounds painful, it is usually painless and cannot be detected until the time of surgery. Clues at the time of surgery might include no sperm or a creamy white fluid from the testicular ends of the vas deferens after the scarred end of the vas deferens has been opened. Sometimes the scar tissue formed after epididymal blowout can be seen in the epididymis.

When such clues are present and reversal is done more than nine years after vasectomy, a *vasoepididymostomy* is commonly performed. In this case, the pelvic or abdominal end of the vas deferens is microsurgically attached to an epididymal tubule above the blockage. This allows sperm to move from the testicle through part of the epididymis and through the vas deferens. A vasoepididymostomy is a much trickier operation than a simple reversal and adds at least half an hour to the procedure. It requires considerable skill and should be undertaken only by physicians who do this on a frequent basis.

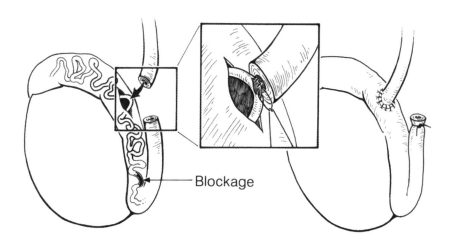

Blockage

An epididymal blowout has scarred and blocked the epididymis. To reverse this vasectomy, the vas deferens is sutured to the epididymis above the blockage in a procedure called vasoepididymostomy. This allows sperm to bypass the epididymal blockage.

The success rate of vasoepididymostomy is pretty good, but it is lower than that for vasovasostomy. Chances are 60 percent that the connection will be open (patent) and around 30 percent for a pregnancy if a vasoepididymostomy is done on both sides.

Sometimes a vasoepididymostomy is needed on one side and only a vasovasostomy on the other. This provides around a 75 percent patency and a 50 percent pregnancy rate, which is between the success rates of vasovasostomies and vasoepididymostomies done on both sides.

Find out whether your surgeon is capable of doing a vasoepididymostomy should the need occur. Remember, the urologist cannot tell whether a vasoepididymostomy is necessary until surgery is in progress. Even during surgery, it may be difficult to determine whether there is epididymal blowout. Many urologists do a vasovasostomy first. If no sperm appears in the ejaculate afterwards, the patient can always go back to surgery for a vasoepididymostomy at a later time.

As a rule, if a man is ten years or more from vasectomy, reversal should be done only by someone who can also do a vasoepididymostomy. There's no sense in wasting time, money, and emotion on a vasovasostomy when the chance of epididymal blowout is high. It's nice to know that, because we can do vasoepididymostomy, there's no time limit on when a vasectomy reversal can be done. And sometimes, even when a vasectomy is long past and epididymal blowout is expected, it doesn't occur. For example, one gentleman came in for a reversal 18 years after a vasectomy. He had divorced and remarried and wanted additional children. He was told of the high chances for epididymal blowout and that he would likely need a vasoepididymostomy. He was quoted a 30 percent pregnancy rate after vasoepididymostomy. In surgery, he had clear fluid with some sperm, indicating he did not have epidymal blowout. Bilateral vasovasostomies were performed, and about four months later he and his wife had a pregnancy.

The complications for vasoepididymostomy are the same as that for vasovasostomy—mainly a slight chance of bleeding, postoperative pain, and infection. If any of these problems develop, contact your physician as soon as possible. Treatment is usually easier when these problems are not ignored.

Alternatives to Reversal

It's a common misconception that sperm can be obtained easily from the epididymis and injected into the partner's uterus to achieve a pregnancy. Indeed, we can remove sperm from the epididymis through a surgical procedure called *epididymal aspiration*. But the procedure results in only a small amount of sperm and requires the use of *in vitro* fertilization (IVF) and sperm injection (ICSI). The drawbacks to IVF are its high cost and relatively low success rate when compared with vasectomy reversal. For these reasons patients with vasectomies are encouraged to consider a reversal before epididymal aspiration with IVF and ICSI. An unsuccessful vasectomy reversal does not preclude attempting IVF and ICSI at a later time.

The Bottom Line

- Vasectomies can be reversed. A reversal requires microsurgical skills and should be performed by a physician who does this procedure on a regular basis (25 cases per year). The overall pregnancy rate is 50 to 70 percent with a 90 to 95 percent chance of sperm in the ejaculate after a traditional vasectomy reversal is performed on both sides.

- Sperm building up in the epididymis after vasectomy may cause epididymal blowout. In this case, a vasoepididymostomy is necessary for reversal. When vasoepididymostomy is performed on both sides, the chances for sperm in the ejaculate are around 60 percent and for a pregnancy, 30 percent.

- The longer a man waits after vasectomy, the greater his chances for epididymal blowout. So don't wait. Call on a qualified surgeon to perform your reversal just as soon as you and your partner decide on it.

8

Impotency

What's up with impotency?

Impotency . . . the very word strikes fear in the heart of most men. Not to be confused with infertility (difficulty in conceiving a child), impotency is the inability to have an erection that is satisfactory for sexual relations. Impotency also is called erectile dysfunction. Though few men readily admit they have a problem with erections, the reality is that impotency affects 10 to 20 million men in the United States on a long-term and significant basis.

Though we tend to think impotency affects only the elderly, it is a problem for many younger patients, even those in their teens. In fact, probably every male has or will suffer from impotency at some point in his life. It may be a short-term problem after a night of heavy drinking, or it may be persistent. The man who suffers from impotency does not suffer alone but has a problem shared by millions. The good news for men with impotency—there's great treatment available!

Anatomy of the Penis and How Erections Occur

Within the penis lie two tubes, or *corpora*. With the penis in the upward or erect state, the corpora lie on top, and the urethra lies on the bottom.

The outer covering of the corpora is of a tough, leatherlike tissue called *tunica albuginea*. Within the corpora is spongy tissue made up of muscle. In the non-erect (*detumesced*) state, blood flows into the spongy tissue through the arteries and immediately flows out the corpora through the veins. With stimulation, the smooth muscle in the corpora relaxes, and the spaces in the spongy tissue enlarge and fill with blood. The swelling of the corporal tissue pinches off the veins and prevents blood from leaving the corpora. Blood going into this relatively closed space fills the corpora like a balloon, causing an erection. Later, with constriction of the muscle, blood leaves via the veins, and the penis becomes limp.

Causes of Impotency

Once it was thought that 80 to 90 percent of men with impotency had psychological causes for their difficulty. It was all in their heads. With increasing knowledge of the physiology of erections, we are able to diagnose more and more physical causes of impotency. We now say that 80 to 90 percent of patients have a physical cause and 10 to 20 percent have a psychological cause for impotency. In the future, as diagnostic methods continue to improve, even more physical causes for impotency likely will be discovered.

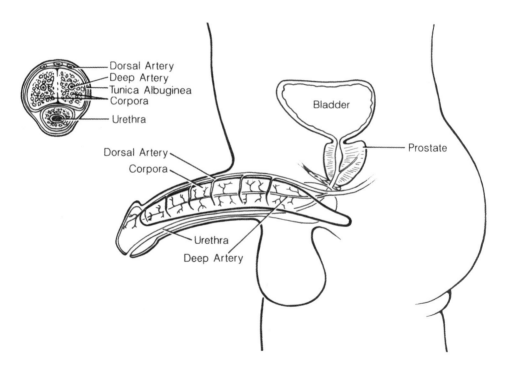

At left is a cross-section of the penis. The urethra is on the bottom, and both erectile chambers, or corpora, are on top. At right, the corpora form a tube that can fill with blood. Half of each erectile chamber is inside the body (there's more to the penis than meets the eye).

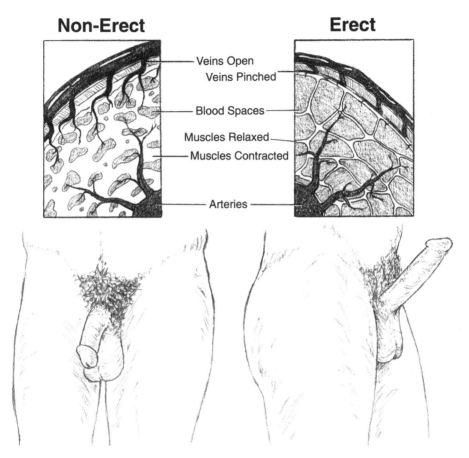

In the detumesced, or non-erect state, the spaces in the corpora are constricted. This allows blood to flow into and out of the penis. With stimulation, the muscle surrounding these spaces relaxes, and the spaces open and fill with blood. The expanded spaces pinch off the veins and prevent blood from leaving the penis. This makes the penis expand, get hard, and after that . . .

There are many classification systems for the causes of impotency. The easiest is to categorize the causes as psychological, neurological, vascular, and other. We will discuss some of the causes of impotency within this framework.

Though the physical reasons for impotency are many, once a man has difficulty with erections, psychological factors often kick in too. In other words, if a man has difficulty performing, the next time he tries to have sexual relations he may recall his previous difficulties. This may cause *performance anxiety*, which may inhibit his erections and cause even more performance anxiety the next time. Most patients with impotency have some problem with performance anxiety. What must be determined is whether this is the major cause or a by-product of impotence. In addition, depression and other psychological problems can affect both erections and sexual drive.

Nerves play an important role in achieving erections. Nerves are the pathways from the brain and spinal cord to the penis; they are involved in releasing chemicals called neurotransmitters. These transmitters relax the smooth muscle in the corpora, which then fill with blood. Therefore, many diseases that affect nerves also affect erections. Probably the most significant neurological disease is diabetes, which can affect blood vessels as well as nerves to the penis. Approximately 50 percent of all diabetic men become impotent after age 50.

Multiple sclerosis, Parkinson's disease, and other neurological conditions that damage nerves can also affect erections. Men who have had the nerves to the penis removed along with their prostates because of prostate cancer often suffer from impotency. Finally, about 10,000 people every year incur spinal cord injuries. Eighty percent are male, and virtually all have difficulty with erections.

Vascular problems, or difficulties with the flow of blood, are detrimental to the extremities. We're talking legs, arms, and penis. As mentioned above, diabetes affects not only the nerves but also the blood vessels that go to the penis. Atherosclerosis, which can cause coronary artery disease, is another major cause of impotency. This disease, affecting the blood vessels that go to the heart, can also affect the blood vessels to the penis. The same can be said for the silent killer, hypertension: high blood pressure may affect the arteries to the penis.

We used to think cigarette smoking only caused lung cancer. Forget it. Cigarette smoking can affect the blood vessels to the penis. About 70 percent of men who smoke 20 cigarettes a day for 20 years or more have blocked penile arteries. Maybe this warning should be put on cigarette packages: "Cigarettes can cause impotency."

Many causes of impotency do not fit neatly into the psychological, vascular, or neurological categories. A common "other" cause of impotency is side effects from medications, especially many of the antihypertensive medications such as beta-blockers and thiazides. Caution: men who are on a medication to control blood pressure may have life-threatening problems if they stop taking it. Controlling blood pressure is more important than the potential side effects of impotency. So if a man on these medications has a problem with erections, he should not stop taking the medication without talking to his physician. Perhaps his doctor can prescribe a medication with less effect on erections or one to help with erections. Other common prescriptions that may adversely affect erections include diuretics, antipsychotics, antidepressants, and antianxiety medications. Again, do not discontinue a medication without a physician's advice.

Problems with hormones can affect erections as well as sexual drive. These include not only low testosterone but also high prolactin (*hyperprolactinemia*) and high or low thyroid hormone levels (*hyperthyroidism* and *hypothyroidism*, respectively). Alcoholism and substance abuse also affects erections. How ironic that alcohol and other drugs can both increase sexual drive and decrease our ability to perform!

Finding the Cause

Keep this in mind: if a man is having difficulty with erections and it's a problem for him or his partner, he should seek help. The only way to get help is to ask for it. Don't be embarrassed when seeking help for impotency, even if the secretary making the appointment or the health care provider is female. Everyone should know that erections are a normal physiological process . . . just like breathing. Half of the population have penises; they are not unique, nor are problems unique. The healthcare provider wants to help. He or she certainly is not thinking of the personal aspects of erections. The healthcare provider, whether nurse, physician, or counselor, is a professional and should provide an atmosphere in which a man is comfortable bringing up any problem. If they do not make the patient feel comfortable, he should seek another provider.

Despite a matter-of-fact approach to erections by most healthcare providers, some people still are embarrassed about the whole process. It's a "hard" topic to discuss. If you know of someone having difficulty with erections who is not seeking help because he doesn't know it exists or is too embarrassed, encourage him to seek help.

Our patient George, a 35-year-old man with a 20-year history of diabetes, had impotency and could have used such help. Even with his history of diabetes, George could not remember ever being asked about his erections. He had had difficulty with erections for at least 15 years because he was too embarrassed to ask about it. He had never been able to have an erection satisfactory for intercourse during this time. Because George had a severe form of diabetes, little evaluation other than a good history and physical examination was needed. After several treatment options were explained, he opted for injection therapy (see the following pages). The appropriate dose resulted in great erections. He now self-injects and is pleased that he is able to have intercourse. It's unfortunate that for 15 years none of his healthcare providers had asked George if he had a problem with erections. If George is you, don't wait to ask for help.

Evaluations for impotency are typically straightforward but may be complex. Most exams begin with a detailed health history. Remember, there are many potential causes for impotency, and most of these surface in a detailed history. The physician asks questions about previous surgeries, medical problems, and current medications, about smoking and alcohol use. Questions specific to erections may include how long there have been problems, whether the problem is getting worse, whether it occurs all the time or only under certain circumstances, and so forth. These matter-of-fact questions deserve matter-of-fact answers.

The physical examination is usually straightforward. The healthcare provider examines the penis for firm areas called *plaques*. The physician also looks for anatomical problems with the penis such as foreskin that cannot be pulled back. Testicles are examined for size and consistency. Small or soft testicles may mean testosterone is low. Usually a rectal exam is done to make sure the prostate is okay. Finally, the examination may include feeling the thyroid gland or checking pulses for adequate blood flow.

Laboratory evaluation varies depending on the philosophy of the particular healthcare provider. Usually blood is drawn to check for the hormone testosterone. Sometimes other hormones such as prolactin are checked. Some physicians order a urinalysis to rule out bladder infection. Laboratory tests usually depend on what is found during the history and physical examination.

Usually a good history and physical examination are enough to determine the causes of impotency. On occasion, additional tests are necessary. For example, a man under age 40 with no apparent cause for impotency requires more testing to figure out what is going on. A description of possible tests follows.

Tests For Nocturnal Erections. Physicians believe that if a man has erections in the middle of the night, when he is sound asleep and in the rapid-eye-movement (REM) stage of sleep, he has no physical or organic problem. In other words, if someone with impotency has firm erections when asleep, his impotency likely is from a psychological cause. If the man does not have good erections in the middle of the night, the cause may be physical. Most patients believe the erections they have when they wake up are the kind of erections they typically have all night. This is not the case. It is the erections a man has when he is sound asleep that are important for diagnosis.

Checking erections in the middle of the night when the patient is sound asleep is called *nocturnal penile tumescence (NPT)* testing. For such testing, patients usually go to a center to sleep overnight two or three nights in a row. Several nights are necessary since during the first night most men are not comfortable in new surroundings and so exhibit abnormal sleep patterns. By the second or third night most patients have more normal sleep patterns. Little bands are placed around the penis to detect the erections. Probes placed on the scalp indicate when a man is in REM sleep. Other monitors check breathing and heart rate. Finding out how often during REM sleep erections occur, how large the penis gets, and how firm, is the goal.

Performing these studies in sleep centers can be expensive ($1,000 to $2,000 per night). For a more reasonable cost, monitors that check erections of men sleeping at home are now available. One of these is the Rigiscan®, a small take-home computer. At bedtime, bands are placed on the penis, and the machine is turned on. In the morning, the machine is turned off, and the bands are removed. This is done three nights in a row, and the machine is returned. The computer shows the number of erections and how large and firm the penis gets in the middle of the night. Though these measurements probably are not as accurate as those taken in sleep centers, they give a fairly good idea of the quality of erections at a fraction of the cost.

NPT testing, in sleep centers or with home monitors like the Rigiscan®, is a great advance over what was used in the past, the old stamp test. For the mere cost of three to five stamps (depending on the size of the penis), physicians wrapped stamps around

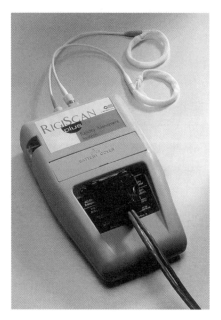

RigiScan Plus Session Graph
Data for Session 1
Sampling Mode: Nocturnal
Session Date: 03/18/95

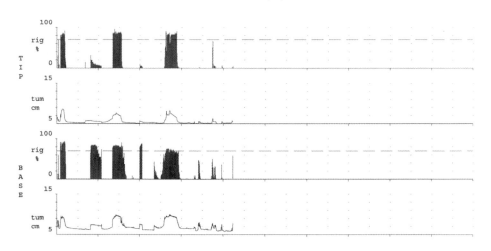

Top, a Rigiscan®. NPT testing with a Rigiscan® or in a sleep lab helps determine whether impotency is due to physical or psychological factors. The machine is strapped to the leg and gauges are attached to the penis. Bottom, the results of one night's sleep: Rigidity and tumescence (swelling) of the tip of the penis are shown on the first two lines. Rigidity and tumescence of the base of the penis are shown on the last two. With four erections at night, this man's penis is in good working order. If he has problems with impotency, it most likely has a psychological cause.

the penis. Their breaking apart during the night supposedly indicated some enlargement during sleep. But simply rolling over in bed could sometimes break the stamps. In attempts to make a more sophisticated "stamp," various bands and cuffs have been developed. A man with no erections does not break the bands. But the test captures only a single moment in time. A break in the band or cuff proves only that there has been one erection that may not have lasted more than a second. So the primary use of this test is to diagnose a severe problem with impotency. If the cuff is placed correctly and does not break, the patient has had no erections at night and is severely impotent. If the band or cuff breaks, the man may or may not have a significant problem, and he still needs further testing.

Evaluating Arteries. A relatively easy screening to check the arteries to the penis is a *penile/brachial index*. In this test, a small blood pressure cuff is placed around the penis. An ultrasound then listens for the penile artery as the cuff is blown up. This is much like obtaining the blood pressure of the penis. The simple office test takes just a few minutes to perform, but it is not very accurate in finding problems with arteries to the penis.

A better test to check the arteries to the penis is *duplex ultrasound*. It uses ultrasound waves to localize the arteries in the penis and check the diameters of the penile arteries, as well as the velocity of the blood entering the artery. A small amount of medication is then injected into the penis to dilate the arteries and relax the smooth muscle of the corpora. This medicine may produce an erection. A tiny needle delivers the medicine, causing little discomfort. The duplex ultrasound then rechecks the diameter of the arteries and the velocity of blood in the penile arteries. Too little increase in the velocity of blood indicates arterial disease. This test also gives an idea as to whether there is a problem with the veins to the penis. It may, for instance, suggest venous leak (see cavernosometry in the following section).

The ultimate test for the arteries of the penis is *arteriography*. A radiologist places a small tube in the femoral artery in the upper thigh, then finds the artery that goes to the penis (pudendal artery) and injects contrast (dye) to show blockages in the penile arteries. A physician performs this test only when considering surgery to unblock the artery or bypass a blockage, usually on young men with a previous history of trauma to the pelvis. Few men with impotency will have this test performed.

Cavernosometry/Cavernosography. In a normal erection, the swelling of the penile tissue pinches off the veins to prevent blood from leaving the penis. With the condition called *venous leak*, the blood goes into the penis, then immediately leaks out of the veins. Typically, men with this condition claim they have firm, initial erections but that they do not last.

Though the history and duplex ultrasound may both suggest venous leak, the definitive test is *cavernosometry*. In this test, the penis is numbed and needles are placed in the corpora (erectile chambers of the penis). Medication injected to dilate the smooth muscle may cause an erection. In cases of venous leak, no erection occurs. Fluid is then pumped into the corpora to simulate the arteries pumping blood into the corpora. Simultaneously, pressure in the corpora is measured. If the corpora cannot hold the fluid and it leaks out the veins, the pressure remains low. If cavernosometry suggests that there is a venous leak, cavernosography is performed. In this test, contrast (dye) injected into the penis helps locate the leaks. Physicians usually do this rare test only when they want to find the exact cause of impotency or fix the leak.

Neurologic Tests. There are numerous, but rarely performed, tests used to check the nerves to the penis. Usually these are done at specialized centers.

Treatment

Remember, effective treatment for impotency is available. In fact, there are more and more new therapies for men with impotence. Typically after diagnosis, the healthcare provider explains various treatment methods, and the patient with the healthcare provider selects the best one. If a particular therapy does not work well, another one usually will.

The Pill. For men with mild impotency, oral medication may be enough. In the past some of these medications, such as Vitamin E, had no specific or known mechanism of action for erections. Others, such as yohimbine or Trazadone®, worked only with mild cases of impotency. Often these medications did not work at all.

Finally, in 1998 the Federal Drug Administration (FDA) approved a pill for the treatment of impotency: sildenafil or, as it is more commonly known, Viagra®. Other oral medications, such as apomorphine (to be marketed by TAP pharmaceuticals as Uprima®) may receive FDA approval around the year 2000. Numerous others are still being developed. These medications have all but revolutionized the treatment of impotency. People are talking about impotency as well as coming in for help now that a pill is available for treatment. These pills are not perfect, however. Virtually all medications have some side effects, and they may not work for everyone.

The first medication available, Viagra®, is taken about one hour before intercourse but not after a big meal. A man who takes it is not going to have an erection just like that. It takes stimulation to make it work. Possible side effects include a hot, red face, headaches, upset stomach, and blurry vision or problems seeing colors. Most men consider these problems mild, and they do not occur often. Still, the man who wants Viagra® should see his physician for an evaluation. This is necessary to find out why he has impotency, to check for other health problems, and to make sure Viagra® is safe for him to take.

One drug interaction known to be harmful involves Viagra® and nitrates. Nitrates, like nitroglycerin, can be taken for chest pain or angina. If a man takes Viagra® and then happens to take a nitroglycerin for chest pain, the combination may lower his blood pressure or even cause death. Death from Viagra® and nitrates is not likely, but it could occur under these conditions. Therefore, check with a physcian before taking Viagra®. Anyone on nitroglycerin or anyone who may need it in the near future should not take Viagra®. If this is you, don't worry. Other great treatments are available, and new oral medications are on the way.

Testosterone Therapy. Testosterone is a male hormone produced by the testis. Its primary effect is to maintain a high level of *libido*, or sexual drive, but it also has a small effect on the penis. For men with low testosterone and mild impotence, testosterone therapy may give better erections. Thus a man who complains of decreased sexual drive may have low testosterone and could benefit from extra testosterone.

One way to get extra testosterone is by injection, usually in the buttocks every two to four weeks. Another way is to wear a body patch. At the time of this writing two types of testosterone patches are available to increase testosterone levels: Testoderm®, made by Alza, and Androderm®, by SmithKline. Both are applied daily. A third way, and most recently introduced, is through a cream. AndroGel®, made by UNIMED, is rubbed into the skin daily. An oral form of testosterone is not used routinely because it can be toxic to the liver.

As with all forms of therapy, testosterone has its side effects. In particular, it can cause the prostate to swell in a way similar to having prostatic hypertrophy (see chapter 10, on BPH). This causes a man to have difficulty with emptying his bladder. It usually shows up as frequent urination both day and night or as difficulty in starting the stream, and the stream may be slow. If this occurs, testosterone injections, patches, or cream probably should stop.

Though testosterone does not cause prostate cancer, if a man develops prostate cancer or has it at the start of testosterone therapy, the hormone will make the cancer grow more rapidly. So men using testosterone injections must have a *PSA* blood test (a molecule in the bloodstream made by the prostate that can give a clue about the presence of prostate cancer) and a rectal examination to check the prostate before therapy begins. Follow-up visits every six months are a must.

Testosterone can also increase the number of blood cells produced, causing thickening of the blood. This is easily diagnosed by drawing blood and checking the blood level in a test called a *hematocrit*. Blood should be obtained once or twice during the course of therapy to make sure that this rare side effect does not occur. In most cases testosterone supplementation causes no problems. For more information on testosterone, see chapter 13, on male menopause.

External Support Sleeve. A new product called ReJoyn® is a soft rubber sleeve that wraps around the penis to give it support for intercourse. ReJoyn® does not give an erection but does allow for intercourse and intimacy. This relatively inexpensive product does not require a prescription and can be purchased at most drugstores.

Vacuum Constriction Device. A vacuum constriction device (VCD) is a relatively new technology developed about ten years ago. It has been a great advancement for patients with impotency. Virtually any man with erectile dysfunction can use it. Many vacuum constriction devices are on the market. Though a prescription is necessary to purchase some VCDs, others are available at pharmacies without prescription.

The devices cost anywhere from $150 to $400. Some companies offer a three-month money-back guarantee. Many come with toll-free numbers, clear instructions, and videocassettes with instructions. (The 1-800 numbers usually do not have people available in the middle of the night, so plan ahead.)

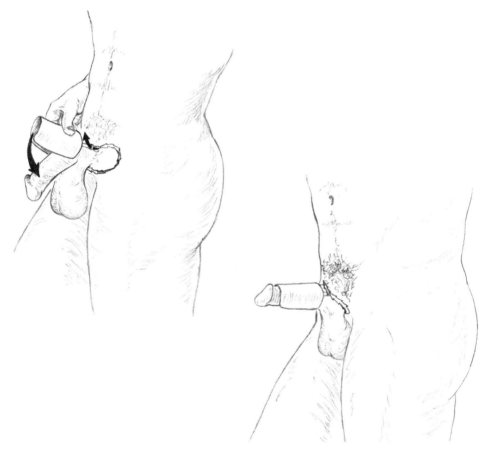

Rejoyn® support sleeve. This soft, rubberlike sleeve makes the penis rigid and allows a couple to have penetration and intimacy.

To use a VCD, the man places the plastic canister or container over the penis. Next he attaches a pump that creates a vacuum in the canister. This pulls blood into the penis and causes an erection within the canister. A thick rubber band or constriction device placed on the base of the penis keeps the blood in the penis. A release valve allows air back into the canister, which then is removed. The man is now ready for intercourse.

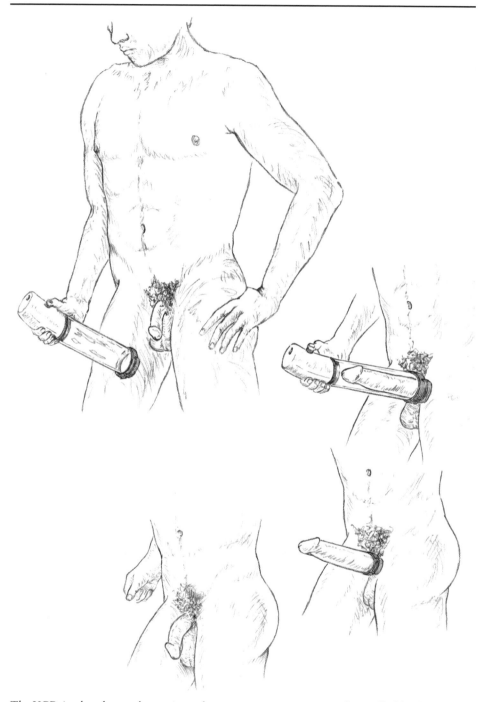

The VCD is placed over the penis, and a pump creates a vacuum that pulls blood into the penis. A constriction ring is rolled onto the base of the penis to keep in the blood. After sex the constriction ring is removed, and the penis goes limp (detumesces).

VCDs are associated with a few minor side effects. Sores or skin erosions may develop if the rubber band is left in place too long. So remove the rubber constriction device after sexual activity (the band should be on for less than 30 minutes). Because the rubber band constricts not only the corpora but also the urethra, the ejaculate may go back into the bladder. Also, patients sometimes complain of coolness and numbness in the penis or of pubic hairs getting caught in the constriction device. Since none of this is serious, and the device is relatively inexpensive, it may be a good solution for the man who does not want pills or more invasive therapy.

The VCD worked well for Mr. Johnson, a 75-year-old who complained of a ten-year history of declining ability to get firm erections. He had had heart problems for years and was on multiple medications. He also had a 20-year history of smoking. Because of multiple causes for his erectile dysfunction, we did not conduct an extensive evaluation. He and his partner chose a VCD from the options explained. After a fair amount of practice and patience, he is now very pleased with the device. Most young, unmarried men do not want to haul around a VCD when they are dating. But for men in stable relationships, it can be a good treatment to start with. If a VCD does not work, other treatment options are available.

Urethral Medications. In 1997 a company named Vivus released MUSE® (medicated urethral suppository for erections). This suppository, smaller than a grain of rice, contains the medication alprostadil, or prostaglandin E1. The medication is put in the urethra via the opening at the tip of the penis with the assistance of a small plastic tube. It does not hurt at all. The penis is held upright until the medication dissolves, in about five to ten minutes. Absorbed into the corporal tissue, the medication helps the blood vessels to open and the penis to fill with blood (an erection occurs). MUSE® is easy to use, convenient (not much equipment is involved), and has fewer side effects than injection therapy (see next section). Lightheadedness and penile pain are potential side effects and the quality of erections tend not to be as good as injection therapy.

Injection Therapy. This therapy is a great example of how understanding the basic science of erections has helped us develop new treatments for impotency. After learning that an erection involves the relaxation of muscles in the corpora of the penis, clinicians hypothesized that injecting medicines to dilate the blood vessels or muscles in the corpora might also cause erections. Shortly thereafter came the advent of injection therapy.

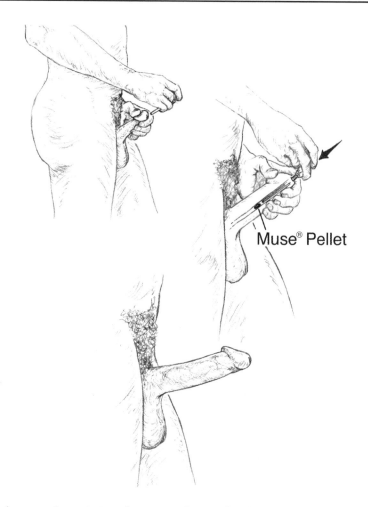

Muse® Pellet

MUSE® is simple to use. Insert it into the penis and press the plunger to force a small pellet of prostaglandin E1 into the urethra. The prostaglandin E1 dissolves and spreads through the penis to give an erection.

With this treatment men inject a small amount of a medication in the corpora that dilates smooth muscle and blood vessels. Commonly used medications are papaverine, phentolamine, or prostaglandin E1, and combinations of these. Until recently the FDA approved these medications only for other uses, not for penile injections, even though they have been used for this purpose for more than ten years. Prostaglandin E1 (Caverject® by Pharmacia UpJohn and Edex® by Schwartz Pharma) has now received FDA approval for use in penile injections. Pharmaceutical companies are seeking approval of other medications for penile injection as well.

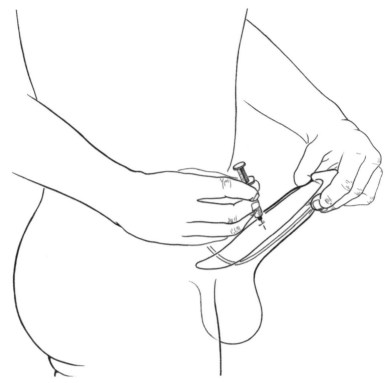

A small (emphasis on small) needle is used to inject medication into the corpora of the penis. The medication spreads through the penis and relaxes the spaces in the corpora, allowing them to fill with blood for an erection. Injection therapy gives a good erection but has mild, potential side effects like scarring of the penis and prolonged erection (priapism).

A tiny syringe with a tiny needle is used to inject medication into the base of the penis. The injection site is held for a couple of minutes. The injections usually give an erection lasting anywhere from ten minutes to two hours. Men can be on injection therapy forever, or they may need it for only a short time to help them over a difficult period in their lives.

Pete, a 25-year-old with impotence, is an example of the latter. He had been married for three years without ever having an erection satisfactory for intercourse. He was embarrassed about his predicament, to state it mildly. His history and physical examination were normal. Using a Rigiscan®, we checked him for nocturnal erections. It showed that he had good erections when asleep. With further questioning, we learned that the couple had a difficult time with the first attempt at intercourse. This led to performance anxiety and even more difficulty on the second attempt. The performance anxiety worsened, and Pete was never able to achieve penetration. He then did what he could to avoid intercourse.

In conjunction with visits to a psychologist, Pete began injection therapy as a temporary help. He easily learned how to inject the medication (papaverine) into his penis to get an erection. The idea was to allow him to achieve penetration so he could "learn" intercourse. After seeing that he could have erections with the injections, he used it once or twice with his wife, then did not need it at all. Recently, his wife became pregnant, and they are happy with their sexual life.

Injection therapy has revolutionized the treatment of erectile dysfunction. It creates a natural erection. Potential side effects include scarring (Peyronie's plaques) and *priapism* (an erection that lasts too long). If an erection lasts more than three hours, call a physician immediately. Though prolonged erection (priapism) sounds great, it's not. Blood left in the penis for more than three hours can cause scarring because the blood is depleted of oxygen. If help is sought immediately, priapism usually is treated easily by injecting medicine into the penis, which causes the smooth muscle to constrict and the penis to become limp. Injection therapy can cause bruising also. With the proper method of injection, however, these side effects are rare. Most important, injections do not hurt because such a small needle is used.

In choosing injection therapy, make sure the healthcare provider has experience with the treatment and can provide proper instruction. In particular, the physician should not start the patient on a large dose but give test doses to find the minimal amount of medication that works well. The physician or nurse should give instruction on how to inject, provide educational materials, and explain what to do should a prolonged erection occur.

Penile Prosthesis. Rods surgically implanted in the penis are *penile prostheses*. The rods make the penis firm enough for a man to have sex. Penile prostheses once had a bad name because they involved surgery and the prostheses frequently failed. With time, prostheses have improved in performance, and the rods give a more natural-looking erection. The failure rate is down to about 15 to 20 percent over a five-year period.

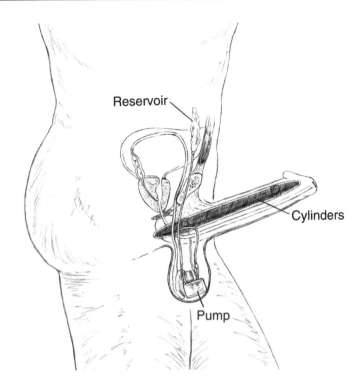

One example of a three-piece penile prosthesis. The cylinders are inserted in the erectile chambers of the penis, the pump is placed in the scrotum, and a reservoir (balloon) with fluid is put in front of the bladder. Here the penis is erect. The release button to make the prosthesis go down is part of the pump in the scrotum. A three-piece penile prosthesis becomes firm when erect and looks soft in the detumesced or non-erect state. It's so natural, it's like the Mercedes-Benz of penile prostheses. The cylinders, reservoir, and usually the pump cannot be seen from the outside.

Prostheses vary from simple to complex. The procedure to put a prosthesis within the erectile chambers (corpora) is relatively easy. It takes anywhere from 30 minutes to two hours depending on the type of prosthesis. Patients are sometimes released that day. Other times they stay overnight for intravenous antibiotics and pain control. They should allow six weeks after insertion before having sex for the tissues around the prosthesis to heal. Then the patient should see his physician for instruction in using the prosthesis.

Not everyone who gets a prosthesis is "old." Bill, age 30, came in with a year-long history of worsening erections. He claimed his penis began to curve upwards and to the left at the onset of his problem. He had two children and came to the appointment with his wife. They appeared to be close and to have a loving relation-ship. On examination we found a plaque, or scar tissue, in his penis. This presumably caused venous leak. Duplex ultrasound showed no evidence of problems with the arteries. Cavernosometry documented venous leak. Bill decided to try surgery to stop the leak, but six months later he still had a problem. After further discussion, Bill elect-ed to have a three-piece penile prosthesis inserted. The operation went well, and Bill is pleased that he is able to have erections.

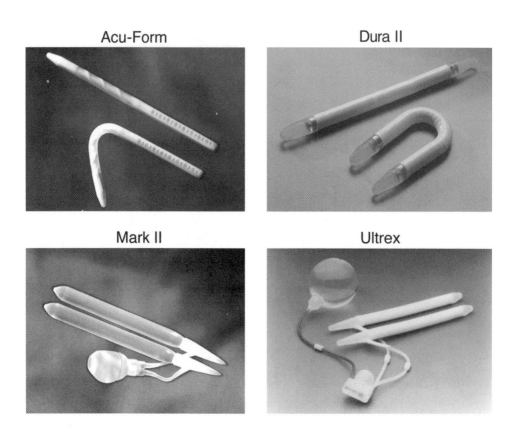

Acu-Form

Dura II

Mark II

Ultrex

Various penile prostheses. Though prostheses require surgery and often an overnight hospi-tal stay, the men who get them by and large like them. The prostheses shown are: (top left) a malleable called an Acu-Form®, (top right) a malleable called Dura II®, (lower left) a two-piece inflatable called a Mark II®, and (lower right) a three-piece inflatable called an Ultrex®.

Side effects of prostheses include malfunction, infection, and pain. If a malfunction occurs, the prosthesis must be replaced. Fortunately, replacement usually is easier than the original insertion. Infection is a serious side effect that occurs in up to 5 percent of recipients. The prosthesis usually must be removed and reinserted at a later time. Occasionally pain is a side effect, but this is rare. Though prostheses require surgery, they usually perform well, and their satisfaction rate is high.

Revascularization and Venous Surgery. For those few men who have a blocked artery to the penis, revascularization is an option. This involves microsurgery. An artery is taken from the abdominal wall and connected to the penile artery. This bypasses the blocked artery. This procedure rarely works for men who have diabetes or who smoke, because they often have multiple blocked sites. The best candidates for revascularization are men who have had trauma causing blockage in a single area of the artery.

Men with venous leak may benefit from venous ligation. In this operation, the veins are tied off to block the blood flow from the veins. This procedure is rarely suggested for men with impotency. Candidates for venous ligation should have no arterial disease. Typically, venous ligation surgery can help for a short time, but venous leak often redevelops over time. This surgery should be done only at specialized centers that deal with impotency.

Remember, while all these therapies help men to have erections, the erections are not completely natural or identical to what they were before impotency developed. Look for improvement but not a perfect cure.

The Bottom Line

- Impotency, or erectile dysfunction, affects about 20 million men in the United States at a given time. Every man likely experiences impotency at some point in his life.

- Erections are a completely normal process, nothing to be embarrassed about. If a man has problems with erection, he should seek help. If he doesn't feel comfortable asking his healthcare provider about impotency, he should find another. One way is to find "Physicians" in the yellow pages and look under the subheading "Impotency."

- Diagnosing the causes of impotency can be simple or complex depending on the circumstances of each case.

- Many effective treatments for erectile dysfunction are available. These include pills, pumps, MUSE, injections, and penile prostheses. Choice of treatment depends on patient preference, the cause of the problem, and how severe the erectile dysfunction. It works best when the patient, his partner, and the healthcare provider decide on a therapy together.

9

Prostatitis

A pain in the butt

Prostatitis is a term commonly used to describe symptoms associated with the prostate, a walnut-sized gland right below the bladder. The major symptom of prostatitis is pain in the bladder, anus, or anywhere between. Though prostatitis may occur at any age, it typically occurs in men in their thirties or older. If a man has recurring urinary tract infections or any of the pains described above, he should see a urologist for evaluation and treatment.

Evaluation for Prostatitis

The physician will want a thorough history of symptoms and complaints. Prostatitis typically causes pain or discomfort in the rectum, pain in the *perineum* (area between the scrotum and anus), *suprapubic* pain (area above the pubic bone, near the bladder), pain with ejaculation, burning with urination, the urge to urinate frequently, the feeling that one cannot completely empty the bladder, testicular discomfort or pain, and general malaise. Other problems associated with the urinary tract, such as kidney stones, problems urinating, and previous surgery to the bladder, prostate, testicles, or kidneys, will also be reviewed to see whether anything else may be causing the current problem.

After obtaining a history the physician will perform a physical examination, particularly a rectal exam to feel the prostate gland. The physician checks for tenderness and the feel of the tissue. Sometimes, the doctor presses hard to get fluid from the gland to come out of the urethra at the end of the penis. This is a prostatic massage; it makes a guy feel like he has to urinate. The fluid collected by prostatic massage is examined under a microscope to see if there is a high number of white blood cells, which may indicate inflammation or infection. The doctor may culture this fluid to see whether it contains bacteria. The rectal exam is not an enjoyable or even comfortable experience, but it usually does not hurt.

Physicians often ask for a urinalysis and a urine culture when checking for prostatitis. On rare occasions they do localization studies to see where an infection originates: the urethra, prostate, or bladder. For these studies, the physician asks the patient to *void* the first few drops of urine in one container, then to start voiding and collect a midstream specimen in a second container. In some cases, after the midstream urine is collected, an ejaculate or fluid from a prostatic massage is obtained for a third culture. Finally, another few drops of urine go into a fourth container.

Depending on the results of the history, physical examination, and cultures, other studies, such as an *intravenous pyelogram*, are obtained. In this x-ray study, contrast (dye) is injected into the veins and excreted from the kidneys. This makes for good pictures of the kidneys. Sometimes *cystoscopy* is performed. In cystoscopy, a telescope is placed into the urethra of the penis, through the prostate, and into the bladder. Though this procedure is uncomfortable, it is a minor test routinely done in the doctor's office.

Causes and Treatment of Prostatitis

After the tests are analyzed, the physician will be able to say whether the patient has prostatitis. What kind he has will determine the treatment. There are, in general, four different types of prostatitis: acute, chronic, nonbacterial, and prostatodynia.

Acute prostatitis usually constitutes an emergency. A history and physical examination clearly will point out this diagnosis. A man with acute prostatitis often has a fever and chills as well as an exquisitely tender prostate. He needs hospitalization for antibiotic treatment. Three to four days of intravenous antibiotics often will cure him, though he'll need to take oral antibiotics for several weeks. If the patient does not respond to intravenous antibiotics in the hospital, the physician looks for a pocket of infection (abscess) in the prostate or for some other cause. Any collection of infection usually needs to be drained.

With chronic prostatitis a man has symptoms of burning with urination and perineal and suprapubic pain but rarely a fever. On examination, the prostate may be slightly tender. For the accurate diagnosis of chronic bacterial prostatitis, bacteria must be cultured from the prostate, a difficult process. Many physicians assume that chronic prostatitis is bacterial even when they have not obtained a culture or when the culture has come back negative.

Chronic prostatitis may be difficult to cure because it is hard to get rid of all the bacteria. When antibiotics are taken for chronic prostatitis, the organism may disappear for a while but then come back. Consequently, men with chronic prostatitis often have symptoms that come and go for a long time.

The treatment for chronic prostatitis usually is to take an antibiotic over a long period, such as one to three months. The important thing is to get a culture showing that there is an organism, then after treatment to get a culture showing it is gone. If an infection does not go away, treatment with a different antibiotic or a longer duration may be necessary. Finally, if a man feels better after antibiotic treatment but the cultured organism keeps coming back, he may be given suppressive antibiotics. This is a low dose taken every day to minimize the infection and the symptoms of prostatitis.

Nonbacterial prostatitis usually is an inflammation of the prostate for which no bacteria are found. This is a frustrating disease because the physician does not know whether it is caused by an organism treatable with antibiotics or if something else is going on. With nonbacterial prostatitis, it is best to start with two weeks of an antibiotic such as erythromycin to find out whether an organism that can cause infection of the urethra, such as chlamydia or ureaplasma, is the cause. Erythromycin is effective against both of these. If this does not work, treatments such as hot tub baths, prostatic massage by the physician, frequent ejaculation, anti-inflammatory agents (such as aspirin), muscle relaxants, or medications to relax the bladder may help.

Prostatodynia usually has the same symptoms as prostatitis, but something outside the prostate is the cause. We don't know the reason, but sometimes the muscles that make up the pelvic floor or the bladder or other muscles outside the prostate may not be working well. Spasms in these muscles can produce the same symptoms as chronic prostatitis or nonbacterial prostatitis.

Treatment for prostatodynia is also difficult and frustrating. Diseases that can mimic prostatodynia include cancer of the lining of the bladder, inflammation of the bladder (interstitial cystitis), and stones in the bladder. The physician should check for these. Medications to relax the bladder neck or the muscle of the bladder and the sphincters may be useful. Again, hot tub baths and anti-inflammatory agents also may give relief. When all else has failed, men with these symptoms should be treated for chronic pain syndrome. Counseling through a pain clinic may be necessary.

The Bottom Line

- Prostatitis is fairly common.

- Cultures are not obtained as often as they should be, and offending organisms or bacteria may not be identified. Make sure cultures are obtained before taking antibiotic treatment.

- If chronic prostatitis is the diagnosis, long-term antibiotic therapy (four to 12 weeks) is the preferred treatment.

- If no organism is found, and if antibiotic therapy is not working, try other treatments. If these treatments fail, seek help for chronic pain syndrome at a pain clinic or elsewhere.

10

Benign Prostatic Hyperplasia
The swollen prostate

Benign prostatic hyperplasia (BPH), commonly thought of as a swollen prostate, is another affliction that nearly all males get if they live long enough. About 50 percent of all men over age 50 have some degree of BPH. This increases to 90 percent of men over 80. About 400,000 men were surgically treated for BPH in the United States in 1990. The good news is that there have been many new medical and surgical advances in the treatment of BPH during the past five years, and many more are around the corner.

Anatomy and Physiology

As urine leaves the bladder, it goes first through the prostate gland. The back of the prostate is located right next to the rectum. As most men know, this allows the prostate to be checked by a rectal examination. Though the prostate gland makes fluid that probably helps sperm survive, its exact function is unknown. Its primary purpose seems to be to give men grief.

About one-third of ejaculate is made up of fluid from the prostate gland. The secretion probably helps sperm move and avoid detection by the female's immune system. Another proposed function of the prostate gland is to help prevent bacteria from getting into the bladder and causing a bladder infection. It acts as a barrier and secretes substances hostile to bacterial growth.

With BPH, the smooth muscle and connective tissue of the prostate grows and causes a partial or complete blockage of urine so that it cannot flow out of the bladder. This blockage of urine is responsible for the symptoms and problems of BPH. In some cases the growth increases the size of the prostate. In others it blocks the channel, but the prostate gland remains small. The surgical treatment of BPH is to remove tissue from the inside of the prostate gland to create a channel (like coring an apple) so that urine can pass through the urethra relatively unobstructed. Medication also may be used to shrink or relax the prostate so urine can more easily pass through the urethra.

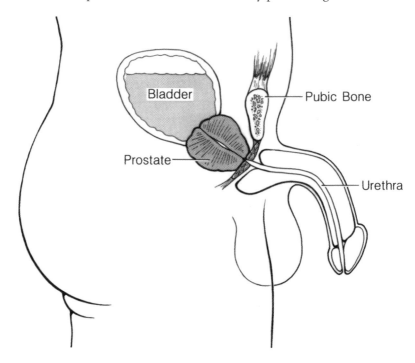

BPH partially blocks the urethra, making urination difficult.

Symptoms of BPH

As mentioned earlier, with BPH the prostate partially or completely blocks the flow of urine as it leaves the bladder and goes through the urethra. This means a common symptom of BPH is decreased urinary flow. Often men with BPH have to urinate more frequently (a symptom called *frequency*). They also may need to get up more often at night to urinate (a symptom called *nocturia*). Some patients with BPH have to get up every 30 to 60 minutes to go to the bathroom, which is disruptive to sleep. Men with BPH also may have difficulty starting the urinary stream. They tend to stand around the toilet and wait and wait and wait until urine eventually comes out. In the most severe cases of BPH, the prostate can be so obstructing that it prevents any urine from being voided. Men with symptoms from BPH are said to have *prostatism*.

Treatment of BPH

If the problems of BPH are severe enough to be bothersome, treatment probably is in order. "The American Urological Association Symptom Index" provides a method of determining the severity of symptoms of BPH. Scores of 8 to 19 indicate a moderate problem and a possible need for treatment. If the score is 20 or above, the man probably has severe problems and definitely should seek help from his physician. Men can take this test themselves to see whether they have prostatism. They also can take it more than once to see how the score changes with time.

American Urological Association (AUA) Symptom Score

Over the past month...,	Not at all	Less than 1 time in 5	Less than half the time	Half the time	More than half the time	Almost always	Total
How often have you had a sensation of not emptying your bladder completely after you have finished voiding?	0	1	2	3	4	5	
How often have you had to urinate again less than two hours after you finished urinating?	0	1	2	3	4	5	
How often have you found that you stopped and started again several times when you urinated?	0	1	2	3	4	5	
How often have you found it difficult to postpone urination?	0	1	2	3	4	5	
How often have you had a weak urinary stream?	0	1	2	3	4	5	
How often have you had to push or strain to begin urination?	0	1	2	3	4	5	
How many times did you most typically get up to urinate from the time you went to bed until the time you got up in the morning?	0	1	2	3	4	5	
					Total of circled numbers:		
				Score:	8-19 = a moderate problem		
					20+ = a severe problem		

An AUA Symptom score of 8 to 19 means a man has a moderate problem with prostatism and may want to undergo treatment for BPH. A score of 20 or more means a severe problem, and the man should seek help from a urologist.

There are other reasons for treating BPH. When a man urinates, he usually empties his bladder completely. Sometimes the BPH obstructs enough that some urine remains in the bladder. A man with this condition has *residual urine*. High residual urine may make him prone to urinary tract infections. Though women often have urinary tract infections because their short urethras make it relatively easy for bacteria to infect the bladder, men typically do not because their urethras are long. Many medical problems (for example, bladder or kidney stones or prostatitis) can cause urinary tract infections in a man, and BPH is one of them. Therefore, if a man gets a urinary tract infection, he likely has a medical problem that needs treatment. Severe blockage may also hurt the kidneys. If the kidneys seem affected, BPH should be treated. Finally, if blockage is severe enough that a man cannot urinate, BPH should be treated.

For moderate cases of prostatism, nonsurgical treatments may be helpful. Recent advances in medicines used to treat BPH are based on the understanding that nerves stimulate alpha receptors in the prostate. The alpha receptors, in turn, cause the smooth muscle of the prostate to contract. These are the same alpha receptors found in the smooth muscle of blood vessels, and they are responsible for high blood pressure, or hypertension.

One way to treat high blood pressure is to block these alpha receptors, thus causing the smooth muscle to relax and the blood vessels to dilate. The same medicines that block alpha receptors in blood vessels can be used to block alpha receptors in the prostate. When the smooth muscle relaxes, the prostate allows urine to pass more easily, and the symptoms of BPH improve. These medications include Hytrin®, Cardura®, and Flomax®, which have been shown to help about one-third of all men with moderate BPH.

Another medication used to shrink the prostate and improve the symptoms of prostatism is Proscar®. This medication prevents the male hormone testosterone from converting into another hormone called DHT (dihydrotestosterone). DHT is the main hormone that causes the prostate to grow. Because a man on Proscar® has lower levels of DHT, his prostate should shrink or at least not grow as much. Proscar® in general does not work as well as alpha blockers in relieving the symptoms of BPH. But it does decrease the bleeding into the urine (hematuria) that sometimes occurs in men with

BPH. In addition, Proscar® can help men who have lots of urine left in their bladders from going into urinary retention (cannot urinate).

Bob, a 50-year-old, had increasing difficulty with urination over one year. He noticed his stream took a while to get going and was weaker once it started. Just a minute after voiding he felt he had to go again (double voiding). He got up about twice a night to urinate. His symptoms bothered him, and he sought help. He was placed on Hytrin®. When he started taking the Hytrin®, he had some lightheadedness when he stood up. He was told that Hytrin® decreases blood pressure and that lightheadedness is a common symptom. After several days the lightheadedness disappeared. A few weeks later Bob noticed a marked improvement in his urinary stream and less urgency at night. He still lacks the stream of a 15-year-old, but it is much better than it was. He gets up only once a night and is happy with his medication.

Men who have bothersome symptoms and do not improve with medical therapy may be good candidates for one of the new, minimally invasive treatments. One of these is transurethral microwave thermotherapy (TUMT). TUMT heats the prostate so that the tissue obstructing the urethra dies. This requires little if any anesthesia and can be done in the office in about two hours. Afterwards, the patient goes home with a catheter, which is removed a few days later. About 75 percent of patients feel their symptoms are significantly relieved after microwave therapy.

Another new therapy is transurethral needle ablation (TUNA) of the prostate. TUNA uses radiowaves to treat BPH. It usually requires some anesthesia (general or spinal). With TUNA, a needle is placed inside the prostate, and radiowaves are used to destroy the tissue blocking the urinary channel. In still another treatment, called Indigo®, a fiber is placed inside the prostate. The light of a laser travels along the fiber destroying tissue. Both TUNA and Indigo® require more anesthesia than TUMT. But TUNA and Indigo® work better on prostates of certain shapes and on very small or large prostates. The size and shape of the prostate, preferences regarding anesthesia, and the physician's experience determine which treatment is best.

If TUMT, TUNA, or Indigo® does not work or the physician feels a more definitive procedure is indicated, *transurethral resection of the prostate (TURP)* is the gold standard for treatment of BPH. But TURP requires anesthesia, a one-or-two-day hospital stay, and more prolonged convalescence. The patient is put to sleep or given spinal anesthesia, and his legs are put up in stirrups. A scope is inserted through the opening of the penis, through the urethra, and into the bladder. A wire loop put through the scope carries electric current that heats the wire loop so that the urologist can shave off pieces of prostate. The chips of prostate are then irrigated out of the bladder and collected for examination by a pathologist to make sure there is no cancer in the tissue. At the end of the procedure, a tube (catheter) that allows urine to drain freely is put into the bladder. Initially, the urine that drains from the bladder is bloody. After a day or two this clears up, and the catheter usually is removed. The newly opened channel should make voiding much easier.

TURP is similar to coring an apple. Though no incision is made in this procedure, it is a significant operation that requires much skill. Blood loss is a potential risk, though rarely is it severe enough to require a transfusion. Another risk is that the fluid used to irrigate the bladder and prostate may be absorbed into the bloodstream. This could overload the heart and dilute important substances in the bloodstream. Finally, with removal of so much prostate tissue, part of the urinary sphincter may be cut. This can result in *incontinence* (leakage of urine) after the surgery. Urologists do this procedure often, however, so these problems rarely occur.

With every TURP, part of the prostate next to the bladder is removed. Because of this, the fluid (semen) from future ejaculations tends to go into the bladder instead of out the penis. This retrograde ejaculation could be startling to a patient not forewarned; he will have an orgasm but see no ejaculate. This generally is not a problem if the man wants to father no more children. If fertility is a concern, discuss this with a physician before undergoing a TURP. If retrograde ejaculation does occur, there are ways of getting sperm from the bladder for insemination in the female partner.

Another surgical treatment for men with BPH who are too sick to undergo TURP or who have a smaller prostate gland, is transurethral incision of the prostate (TUIP). In this procedure a scope is placed through the penis, and an incision is made from the bladder through the floor of the prostate. This simply opens up the prostate more to allow urine to pass through more easily. No removal of prostatic tissue is involved, so results may not be as good as with a TURP. Nevertheless, TUIP is useful for men with small obstructing prostates and for those who need a shorter, safer procedure.

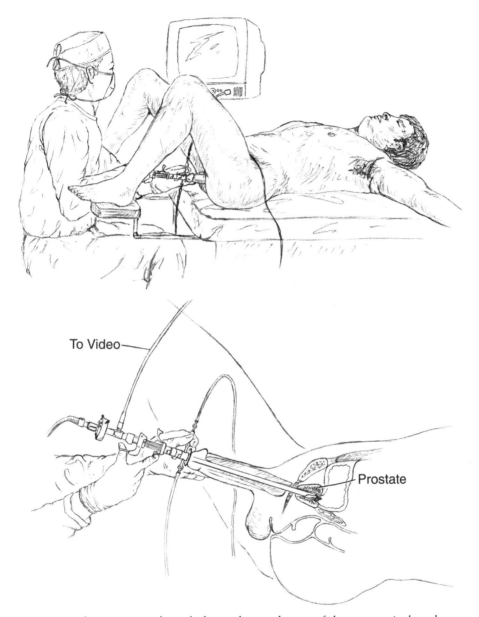

In a TURP, a telescope is put through the urethra, and some of the prostate is shaved out to make the channel larger. This allows urine to pass more easily.

For men who have large prostates, TURP can result in much blood loss and absorption of fluid. These patients need a *simple prostatectomy*. A small incision is made in the lower abdomen and in the bladder or right over the prostate, so that the swollen part of the prostate can be seen and removed. A simple prostatectomy is different from a *radical prostatectomy*, in which the entire prostate is removed as treatment for prostate cancer (see chapter 11, on prostate cancer).

The problem with a simple prostatectomy is that it involves an incision, which makes the recovery time longer. It is safer than a TURP, however, for men with large prostates. Such was the case with Richard, a 65-year-old who noticed over 30 years a marked worsening of his urinary stream. He felt he could urinate only by sitting on the toilet. He got up every hour at night to urinate. He was cranky and crabby because of this, and his spouse thought he was sleep-deprived.

Richard's physician found that he had a very large prostate gland. He underwent a simple prostatectomy, and the swollen part of his prostate was removed. A week later the catheter was removed, and his stream was much better. Richard had severe BPH; the prostate was causing major problems in his lifestyle and sleeping patterns. Though he needed surgical treatment, he had no complications and significantly improved.

Only the swollen part of the prostate is scraped or shelled out in a TURP and simple prostatectomy. The rest of the prostate gland remains in place. Prostate cancer can develop in the gland remaining. For Sam this was a problem. Sam was a 55-year-old who had noticed a decreased flow of stream for two years. He got up frequently at night to urinate, and he voided every hour during the day. After seeing a physician, he underwent a TURP. He could pass his water more easily afterwards and was happy with the procedure.

After recovery, Sam did not see his physician for three years. Then he went in for a routine physical. A rectal examination showed a hard nodule on his prostate. This surprised him as he thought his prostate had been removed with the TURP. It turned out cancer had developed in the part of the prostate left behind. He underwent a radical prostatectomy, in which the entire prostate was removed. Presumably cured of prostate cancer, he continued to do very well.

Remember, with a simple prostatectomy or a TURP, part of the prostate remains and a man remains at risk for prostate cancer. Men who have these procedures should still have their prostates checked annually for cancer.

Recently, lasers have been used to destroy prostatic tissue and open channels for urination. As with TURP, the patient is put to sleep or given spinal anesthesia. A scope is placed through the penis to the prostate. Lasers are used to burn the prostate tissue. Afterwards, a catheter is put into the bladder and left there for several weeks. Laser prostatectomy tends to be safer than TURP because there is less blood loss. But the catheter can irritate the bladder, and many patients experience pain and an urgency to urinate during the weeks the catheter is left in. A laser prostatectomy is reasonable treatment for a small prostate, whereas TURP can be done with larger prostates. The patient and physician should decide together whether laser prostatectomy or TURP is best.

The exact treatment depends on the severity of the symptoms, the overall health of the patient, and the size of the prostate gland. If one therapy, such as medication, does not work, another may give better results. Sometimes after treatment such as TURP, the prostate tissue grows back. Other times, the swollen part of the prostate is removed and a channel opened, but the symptoms of BPH remain. This may occur because blockage of the urinary stream has damaged the bladder and its nerves. Urologists who specialize in treating BPH can help guide the man with this condition to the best therapy.

The Bottom Line

- BPH affects millions of men in the United States. Nearly every man develops BPH if he lives long enough.

- Symptoms of BPH, caused by a partial or complete obstruction of the urethra by the growing prostate, include decreased flow of urine, voiding frequently during the day and at night, increasing difficulty starting the stream, straining to void, and a feeling after urination that the bladder is not empty.

- Treatments for BPH include many medical and surgical therapies. If one method does not work, another usually will.

- Both TURP and simple prostatectomy leave part of the prostate in place, which may develop prostate cancer. Men who undergo treatment for BPH should continue annual screening for prostate cancer.

11

Prostate Cancer
When the gland becomes deadly

Many people think that only older men get prostate cancer. Many also believe that treatment is not necessary because men with prostate cancer are more likely to die of something else before the cancer gets them. However, it is increasingly clear that prostate cancer can affect men of all ages. It is responsible for the deaths of about 40,000 men in the United States every year. In fact, prostate cancer is the most common cancer in men. Though we have made many advances in the past decade in diagnosing this cancer, many aspects of the disease, especially treatment, remain controversial. In this chapter, we look at who gets prostate cancer, how it typically presents, and what can be done about it.

The Prostate Gland

As discussed previously, the prostate gland is the shape and size of a walnut. It is located at the base of the bladder and makes up the first part of the urethra through which urine goes after it leaves the bladder. The prostate is made up of glands, smooth muscle, and connective tissue (like tendons and cartilage). Glands in the prostate secrete the fluid that is a large part of an ejaculate. The back of the prostate gland, where prostate cancer frequently develops, rests right next to the rectum. This is why rectal examinations are important in helping to diagnose prostate cancer.

Who Gets Prostate Cancer?

Though prostate cancer can occur in men of all ages, it is most common in older men. In fact, it has been said that men who live long enough will get prostate cancer. Up to 80 percent of all men in their nineties show some evidence of prostate cancer.

This data is based on autopsy studies in which prostates examined under a microscope showed minute areas of prostate cancer. We call this "clinically insignificant prostate cancer." It reminds us that most of these men have no symptoms of prostate cancer and do not die from the disease. Nevertheless, 1 to 2 percent of men over age 45 have prostate cancer that can be detected by a rectal examination or a blood test. These cancers have the potential to spread and cause problems, including death. In fact, 20 to 25 percent of men with clinically detectable prostate cancer ultimately die from the disease. The younger you are, the less likely you are to have clinically detectable prostate cancer, but the disease can affect men of any age.

Mike was an athletic, young-looking 48-year-old who was being evaluated for male infertility. He and his partner had been trying to have a child for several years. There was nothing remarkable in his history. As part of his workup, Mike had a rectal examination. He had a slightly firm area on the left side of his prostate that easily could have been dismissed. To be on the safe side, we ordered a transrectal ultrasound (TRUS).

Transrectal ultrasound uses an inch-wide probe, placed in the rectum, to look at the prostate with ultrasonic waves (not radiation). This exam is mildly uncomfortable but does not hurt. Using TRUS, we found an area that looked suspicious for prostate cancer. A biopsy of the area was immediately taken during the TRUS. Because of Mike's age and health, we thought the suspicious area probably was nothing to worry about. But the pathology report returned a week later showing prostate cancer. His focus had to change abruptly from trying to conceive to coping with and treating a life-threatening prostate cancer. Within two weeks, Mike's prostate, with the cancer contained in the gland, was removed. He recovered from surgery and is being followed carefully by his urologist.

Though prostate cancer is common worldwide, it seems particularly prevalent in the United States, England, and Sweden. In the United States, African Americans have the highest incidence of developing and dying from prostate cancer. The cause is debatable. There may be a genetic predisposition to contracting a more aggressive prostate cancer. Or there may not really be an increased incidence of prostrate cancer, but because of less access to early screening and good healthcare, prostate cancer in African Americans is not detected and treated as early as it should be.

Besides race, there are many other risk factors for developing prostate cancer. Increased dietary fat may contribute to getting prostate cancer. There also may be a genetic predisposition. The more blood relatives with prostate cancer and the younger the relatives when diagnosed, the greater a man's chance of getting it too. There are probably many other factors, such as environmental causes, but we don't know much about them yet. Some studies have shown a link between having a vasectomy and getting prostate cancer, but more-recent studies dispute this. Men who have vasectomies probably are more health-conscious and more likely to see their physicians. Therefore, if they have prostate cancer, it's more likely to be diagnosed.

What Are the Symptoms of Prostate Cancer?

A man may have absolutely no symptoms and still have prostate cancer. He can be feeling fine, urinating normally, appear to be in great health, and yet have prostate cancer. This is why, starting around age 50, men should be checked periodically for this disease. Men with a family history of prostate cancer and African Americans should consider screening at age 40.

Some men with prostate cancer have symptoms of prostatism. These men have a partial obstruction of the prostatic urethra and difficulty with urination. They urinate frequently during the day, may get up several times at night, and have difficulty starting the stream. The signs and symptoms of prostatism are not necessarily present in someone with prostate cancer. A man with prostate cancer may present with no symptoms, some symptoms, or all the symptoms of prostatism.

Blood in the urine (hematuria) is another sign that, on occasion, indicates prostate cancer. Sometimes the blood is visible, making the urine red. Other times the blood is microscopic and is picked up only through urinalysis. Finally, though hematospermia (blood in the semen) usually disappears after one or more ejaculations, it also may be a sign of cancer of the prostate.

Sometimes prostate cancer has spread and presents as symptoms common to any widespread disease. These symptoms include night sweats, changes in appetite, weight loss, and just "not feeling well." If the cancer has spread to the bone, it can cause bone pain.

The possible signs and symptoms of prostate cancer are many, but prostate cancer may occur without any at all. This is why yearly exams are important!

The Routine, Possibly Lifesaving Checkup

Just as women have yearly exams for breast and cervical cancer, men should have their prostates examined on a regular basis. Exactly how often men without symptoms should be checked is controversial because of insurance issues. But for an individual, figuring out how frequently and by what means the prostate should be examined is relatively easy.

Though prostate cancer can strike in the early forties, this is uncommon. Therefore, the American Cancer Society recommends a rectal examination every year starting at age 50 in men who have at least a ten-year life expectancy. Though a rectal examination is not the most sensitive way to detect prostate cancer, it is certainly the easiest, least expensive, and most painless. There is no excuse to forego a rectal examination. It should be part of the annual physical examination every man undergoes to maintain good health.

There is some controversy as to whether all men should have their prostate specific antigen (PSA) checked and at what age they should start. PSA is a protein produced by the prostate that is found in blood. PSA levels may increase in males who have BPH or inflammation or infection of the prostate (prostatitis), as well as in those who have prostate cancer. An elevated PSA level does not *necessarily* mean a man has prostate cancer, but it does raise suspicions for it. PSA is a simple blood test costing about $50 to $75. Medicare now pays for an annual PSA level, with some restrictions, for its beneficiaries.

PSA detects at least one-third of prostate cancers previously undetected by rectal examination alone, and it detects them at an earlier stage. This results in treating the cancer when it is potentially more curable. All men should have the test done regularly after age 50.

Some argue that if every male between age 50 and 70 had a PSA level done every year, it would cost the U.S. insurance industry about a billion dollars annually. But how many lives would be saved? Studies in the works, some sponsored by the National Institute of Health, may provide a few answers. Until then, we can only recommend to others what we would want done for ourselves—that a PSA level be obtained each time a man goes in for his yearly physical (including rectal) examination, starting at age 50. Tailor this general rule to the individual. African-American men and men with a family history of prostate cancer should begin at age 40. And they should do it more often, perhaps even every six months.

In the past, if there was suspicion of prostate cancer such as a firm area on the prostate on rectal examination, the patient was put to sleep with general anesthesia to have a biopsy taken. Nowadays, with transrectal ultrasound (TRUS) and the *biopsy gun*, a biopsy of the prostate is an easy and relatively pain-free procedure performed in most clinics. TRUS uses sound waves to identify areas suspicious for prostate cancer that may not be felt on rectal examination.

The biopsy gun, a cylinder used to hold and guide a needle to the suspicious area, is used in conjunction with TRUS to obtain a prostate biopsy. The needle is passed through the TRUS probe, and ultrasound guides the needle to the exact area to biopsy. A spring in the biopsy gun, released by a trigger, shoots the needle into the prostate gland so quickly that the procedure is virtually pain-free. Several biopsies of the prostate in both suspicious areas and nonsuspicious areas are usually obtained. The procedure takes about 15 minutes, and the patient goes home. A pathologist reads the biopsy results within a week.

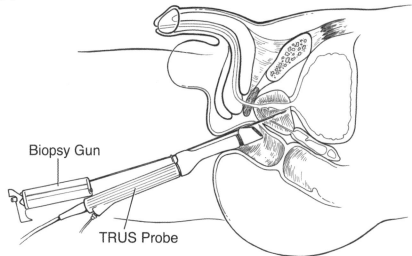

Biopsy Gun

TRUS Probe

A transrectal ultrasound (TRUS) probe is put into the rectum to look at the prostate. Transrectal ultrasound can measure the size of a prostate, identify areas suspicious for cancer, and direct a biopsy gun. This is an uncomfortable procedure, but it doesn't hurt.

It's Cancer—What Happens Next?

If prostate cancer is detected, the big question is whether it has spread beyond the prostate. Sometimes a good rectal examination or TRUS can answer this. More often than not, other tests are necessary. Prostate cancer tends to spread to the pelvic lymph nodes and to bone. If it metastasizes (spreads) to bone, it usually goes to the pelvis or spine. So the physician may order a *bone scan* for a man just diagnosed with prostate cancer.

For this test, a mineral-like substance that tends to go to bone is injected in the veins. The substance is attached to an isotope that emits a low level of radioactivity, less than in a chest x-ray. People with cancer in their bones may show increased absorption of the radioactive substance in the diseased area. But increased activity on a bone scan does not necessarily mean prostate cancer. It could be from some other disease or a previous fracture. Further, the lack of increased activity does not necessarily mean that prostate cancer has *not* gone to the bone. Nevertheless, the bone scan gives a pretty good idea of whether cancer has spread to bone.

If the PSA level is low, chances are the prostate cancer has not gone to bone, and many physicians do not bother to obtain a bone scan in such cases.

Physicians can also use a CT scan to see whether prostate cancer has spread. With a CT scan, the man lies down, and cross-sectional x-rays are obtained of the pelvis. These x-rays provide images like slices of a loaf of bread. The images give some idea of whether the prostate cancer has spread to the lymph nodes, which are small, round bodies in which fluid, white blood cells, bacteria, and cancer can accumulate. CT scans are not a sensitive way of detecting spread to the lymph nodes, however, so most physicians use this test only in special circumstances.

Sometimes physicians use other means for finding out whether prostate cancer has spread. Some use a new radiological test called Magnetic Resonance Imaging (MRI) to see whether prostate cancer has spread beyond the prostate or to the pelvic lymph nodes, or to confirm abnormalities on the bone scan. The physician decides which tests are important to get based on information from the history and physical exam.

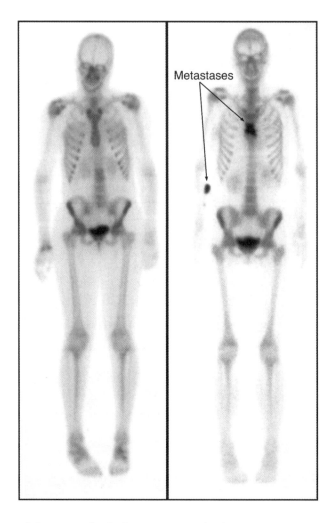

Metastases

The bone scan at left is normal. The bone scan at right shows prostate cancer that has gone (metastasized) to bone.

Treatment of Prostate Cancer

Two methods are used to treat localized prostate cancer: radical prostatectomy and radiation therapy. These treatments are done with hope of a cure. If the checkup shows the cancer already has spread outside the prostate, there is virtually no chance of a complete cure with either method. Furthermore, if a man with prostate cancer likely will not live ten more years because he is in poor health or of advanced age, he should not undergo radical prostatectomy or radiation therapy to the prostrate. This is because prostate cancer tends to grow and spread slowly. A man of 70, or some physicians say 75, is more likely to die of a heart attack, stroke, or some natural cause other than the prostate cancer. Neither should a man under 70 with significant health problems, such as severe diabetes, undergo a radical prostatectomy or radiation therapy.

Don't despair if you fit one of these categories. Remember, the cancer is likely to grow slowly. The growth may be slowed even more through hormonal therapy (see "Other Treatments," later in this chapter). How big the prostate cancer is, whether it appears to be slow-growing (a low-grade cancer) or fast-growing (a high-grade cancer), and your age and overall health must be considered in determining the therapy of choice. Often, the best course is not clear, so be sure to have a good conversation with a physician who knows about prostate cancer. A urologist who specializes in this disease will have the most information. But even among urologists there is sometimes controversy on how to treat prostate cancer. Don't hesitate to get a second opinion if you have any questions about the best course.

Radical Prostatectomy. Let's get back to the man who is younger than 70 and relatively healthy except for his prostate cancer. While there is still some controversy over the best form of treatment, most physicians who treat prostate cancer believe that a radical prostatectomy is optimal for curing this disease. Radical prostatectomies are performed by urologists.

An enema or light bowel prep frequently is given before a radical prostatectomy. The prostate is close to the rectum, and if the rectum is accidentally injured during surgery, it will be easier to fix if it's clear. General anesthesia is usual, but some patients are given epidural anesthesia. This is done by injecting local anesthesia with a needle into the lower back. The anesthesia dulls the nerves and numbs the lower half of the body.

After anesthesia is given, an incision is made from the umbilicus (belly button) to the pubic bone right above the penis. The lymph nodes in the pelvis are then sampled. If any of the lymph nodes are suspicious for prostate cancer, they are sent to a pathologist for immediate examination. If the pathologist detects prostate cancer, the operation often is stopped because the chance of cure by surgery is slight. Some urologists, however, continue the surgery if the cancer has spread only to the lymph nodes, because they feel some benefit to the patient may result. Regardless of whether the operation continues or is stopped, other therapy, such as hormonal treatment, may be given.

Assuming that the pelvic lymph nodes show no cancer, the prostate is removed and the bladder is reattached to the remaining part of the urethra. Drains to prevent the collection of blood and lymph are then placed in the pelvis. A catheter (tube) is inserted through the urethra and penis into the bladder. The entire procedure takes about three hours. Afterwards, the patient stays in the hospital for three to seven days. He usually goes home with the catheter in place; the urologist removes it in a week or so.

A radical prostatectomy is a major operation; it is usually safe when done by an experienced surgeon. The most common complication is impotency. In many cases the man will not be able to get an erection after a radical prostatectomy. This is because the nerves and blood vessels that control erections are located along the prostate and are easily injured during the procedure.

In the early 1980s Patrick Walsh, M.D., and his associates at Johns Hopkins University developed a nerve-sparing radical prostatectomy that is now commonly performed by most urologists. In select patients, the prostate can be removed and the nerves spared. Many of these men will not become impotent. The younger the man and the better his erections before the operation, the greater the chance his erections will be preserved. If the physician believes that cancer could be left behind, however, the nerves won't be spared. The point of surgery is to remove all of the cancer from the patient.

As mentioned above, impotency is a side effect of radical prostatectomy for some men. Depending on the age of the patient, how advanced the cancer is, and whether the surgeon does a nerve-sparing radical prostatectomy, the rate of impotency ranges from 20 to 90 percent. There is new evidence that artificially creating an erection soon after a prostatectomy with either a vacuum constriction device (VCD) or injection therapy delivers oxygen to the penis and improves the likelihood of natural erections returning later. Nevertheless, many patients undergoing radical prostatectomy will not have good erections afterwards. Given the advent of vacuum suction devices, injection therapy, and high-quality penile prostheses, patients should not be overly concerned about impotency.

The next-most-common serious complication is incontinence, the leakage of urine. Most patients have some incontinence immediately after the catheter is removed. In the majority, the incontinence resolves within a year of surgery, and the man can control his urine again. In about 5 percent of patients, incontinence persists and is a serious social problem. Treatment for incontinence includes Kegal exercises (contracting the muscles around the anus to build up the muscles around the bladder), collagen injections to narrow the urethra, inflatable sphincters placed around the urethra, mechanical devices to obstruct the urethra, and devices for collecting urine including padding, such as Depends®.

Another complication is urethral stricturing, a narrowing of the urethra. This occurs in about 10 percent of patients who undergo radical prostatectomy. Strictures usually occur in the area where the bladder is reattached to the urethra. Any one of several methods, depending on the severity of the stricture, may be used to treat it. In some cases the narrowing can be stretched or dilated. In others it must be incised (cut) by a knife or laser to open it up. Other complications, such as rectal injury during surgery, are possible but not common with radical prostatectomy.

Radiation Therapy. Radiation therapy can be given as "external beam" therapy. This is radioactivity aimed in controlled amounts at the prostate. It is useful for treating men in poor health who are not candidates for radical prostatectomy. Sometimes radiation therapy is used for patients with part of a tumor remaining after radical prostatectomy. A radiation oncologist administers radiation therapy multiple times for a certain number of doses.

People commonly think of radiation therapy as not having side effects. Actually, side effects from radiation include impotency in about 20 percent, incontinence in 1 percent, injury to the rectum in about 2 percent, and lymphedema (swelling of the legs) in about 10 percent of patients.

Another use of radiation therapy is for patients who have prostate cancer that has metastasized or gone to bone. In these cases, the patient may have pain in the bone that is being invaded by prostate cancer. In other cases, prostate cancer invading the spine may cause collapse of the spinal column and nerve damage. In these cases of bone fracture or pain because of metastasis, radiation therapy can help to shrink the cancer and decrease bone pain. But it will not rid the bone of prostate cancer completely.

Another new form of radiation therapy is radioactive seed implant. With this method of treating prostate cancer, tiny radioactive seeds are planted directly into the prostate. These seeds are about the size of rice grains. Using TRUS to guide placement, the urologist uses small needles to insert the seeds into the prostate through the perineum, an area between the scrotum and the rectum. Though there is no incision or cutting, because needles are used to place the radioactive seeds, either spinal or general anesthesia is given.

The benefits of radioactive seed implantation, which is an outpatient treatment, include a higher concentration of radiation directly to the cancer, quicker recovery time, and less chance of side effects like incontinence and impotency. Disadvantages include the limited number of physicians trained in seed implantation, the common side effects of frequency or urgency to urinate, and the limited information on rates of complication and long-term success. More and more physicians are learning how to do this treatment, which may well turn out to be a good alternative to surgery (radical prostatectomy) in selected patients.

Other Treatments

If prostate cancer has spread outside the prostate into surrounding tissue, lymph nodes, or bone, the chance of cure is small. But we have outstanding ways to treat symptoms and problems related to the spread of prostate cancer.

If the local spread of prostate cancer blocks the flow of urine into the bladder or causes bleeding or pain, radiation therapy may be helpful. In addition, as discussed above, radiation therapy may help to alleviate localized bone pain from metastasis. If prostate cancer blocks the urethra and causes difficulty with passing urine, a transurethral resection of the cancer may help. In this situation, general or spinal anesthesia is given, and a tube is passed through the urethra and the penis to the prostate. The surgeon uses a loop with electric current to cut a channel in the prostate cancer, just as with a TURP for BPH. This relatively easy procedure takes 30 to 60 minutes to perform, and an incision through the skin is not necessary. The procedure opens a channel so that urine easily can pass through.

In about 80 percent of cases, prostate cancer is dependent on testosterone and other androgens; in other words, the prostate cancer needs testosterone to grow. If testosterone is removed, the cancer shrinks but does not go away completely. Therefore, removing testosterone may relieve or reverse symptoms in men with prostate cancer that is blocking the urethra, causing bone pain, or just causing them to feel weak. In fact, there is some evidence that men with no symptoms from their prostate cancer have a slightly better survival rate when treated early with removal of testosterone.

Testosterone may be decreased in several ways. In the past, many patients took estrogen, but because of serious side effects like heart attacks and strokes, this therapy is no longer in vogue. A method still used today is bilateral *orchiectomy*, the removal of the testicles, a simple and quick procedure. A modification of orchiectomy is sub-capsular orchiectomy, in which only the tissue that produces testosterone is removed from the testicle. The capsule of the testicle is left in place. The patient appears to have testicles remaining, though all the testosterone and sperm-producing material has been removed. The main disadvantage of removing the testicles is that it is permanent and there is no possibility of conceiving more children in the future. This usually is not a major concern for men who have prostate cancer. Still, the loss of the testicles has a significant psychological effect on some.

Another method of decreasing testosterone is by taking a gonadotropin-releasing hormone *(GnRH) analog*, such as Lupron® or Zoladex®. This medication is injected under the skin, usually once every three months. Finally, there are several antiandrogens that block the effects of testosterone. These oral medications include Eulexin®, Casodex®, and Nilandron®. Sometimes GnRH analogs are combined with antiandrogens to make sure no testosterone stimulates the prostate cancer. Downsides to GnRH and antiandrogen therapies are that men must remember to take them regularly and that over the long run they are expensive.

A side effect of all of the therapies that decrease testosterone—orchiectomy, antiandrogens, and GnRH analog—is hot flashes. Hot flashes are waves of warmth that sweep over the body, usually starting with the head. They last a few seconds and may occur several times a day. If hot flashes bother you, talk to your physician about medications that can help decrease them. Lowering testosterone also diminishes a man's libido (urge to have sex). For some men (and partners) this side effect is a problem; for others it's no big deal. In addition, long-term hormonal therapy may cause osteoporosis.

The Bottom Line

- The incidence of prostate cancer increases with age, but it can affect younger men, including those in their forties. In younger men, prostate cancer tends to progress rapidly. Every male over age 50 should be checked for prostate cancer every year by a rectal examination, and by drawing a PSA level. If you are an African American or have a family history of prostate cancer, start the checkups around age 40 and have them more often.

- We recommend radical prostatectomy if prostate cancer is discovered early and the man is expected to live another 10 to 15 years (in general, if he is relatively healthy and under age 70). The implantation of radioactive seeds in the prostate is often an alternative to radical prostatectomy.

- Serious side effects of radical prostatectomy include impotency and incontinence. Both can be treated effectively.

- If the prostate cancer has spread, hormonal treatment may help to control the disease by decreasing or blocking the effects of testosterone.

- Many questions surround the treatment of prostate cancer. For instance, what treatment should follow radical prostatectomy if some tumor is left behind? Should the patient receive radiation therapy, hormonal therapy, or wait until problems develop? And what if prostate cancer spreads to the lymph nodes or bone, but the man has no symptoms? Should the patient receive hormonal therapy early and risk hot flashes and decreased libido? Or should he wait for symptoms to appear? We suggest that every patient seek several opinions and make the decision that suits him best.

12

Male Baldness
For the folliclely challenged

There's more to baldness than meets the eye. Men have different types of hair loss of differing causes, each calling for different treatments. Though we focus here on the most common cause, male-pattern baldness, understanding some other causes of baldness may have important medical implications for a man.

A person's hair does not grow all at the same rate and time. At any particular time, about 90 percent of hair follicles in the head are in a growth phase, called *anagen*, while 10 percent of hair follicles are in a resting phase, called *telogen*. Hair follicles in the growth and resting phases intermingle. Anagen follicles grow for up to three years, whereas telogen follicles rest for about three months. A new (anagen) hair follicle begins to grow under each resting follicle. As this occurs, the old hair falls out. Men frequently describe these hair fibers as "clubbed," as if they fall out by their roots. You may shed a hundred of these old hair fibers every day.

Male hormones, called androgens, are one of several factors controlling hair growth. The male hormone testosterone is converted in tissues to another hormone called dihydrotestosterone (DHT). DHT is the principal hormone thought to control hair growth. In fact, it shortens the growth (anagen) phase. Lots of DHT in the scalp means less hair growth.

Male-Pattern Baldness

Many men are destined or programmed to become bald as they age. This pattern of male baldness is somehow related to androgens. Males who are castrated before puberty and therefore lack most male hormones, do not suffer from male-pattern baldness. This radical therapy for baldness is not recommended for most men! There is also a genetic component to male-pattern baldness. We think the trait is autosomal dominant, which means only one copy of the gene from one parent is enough to cause baldness. Many people believe that if your mother's father is not bald, you will not be bald either, but that is a myth. Other, currently unknown, factors also may influence the rate and extent of male-pattern baldness.

Male-pattern baldness tends to begin in the lateral frontal areas and over the vertex, the topmost part of the scalp. It may begin in the midteens, but usually the onset is later. A man may lose a significant amount of hair before he or others notice a change.

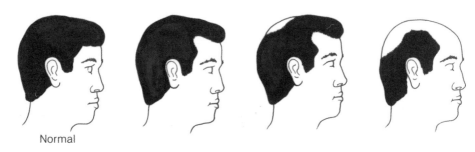

Normal

The progression of male-pattern baldness (from bad to worse).

Treatment for Male-Pattern Baldness

In the opinion of the authors (particularly the bald one), no great medical treatments for male-pattern baldness yet exist. But several medications may help some men with this problem.

Probably the most common medication is topical minoxidil (Rogaine®). This substance, rubbed or sprayed into the scalp, increases the growth (anagen) phase of hair. The original formula of 2 percent minoxidil works in about one-third of men. Its main side effects are itching of the scalp and headaches. You can now buy without a prescription a 5 percent solution of minoxidil called Rogaine Extra Strength®. The 5 percent solution provides nearly 50 percent more hair growth than the 2 percent minoxidil, but its side effects may be more common. Minoxidil used early in adult life may prevent hair loss.

Hair growth resulting from minoxidil often has a texture different from the original hair. When treatment with minoxidil stops, the hair that has grown because of the medication usually falls out. So if you want to use minoxidil for hair growth or to stop hair loss, plan on long-term application, which may be costly.

While minoxidil is applied to the scalp, a new medication called finasteride is taken orally. Finasteride, described in chapter 10 on benign prostatic hyperplasia (trade name is Proscar®), is sometimes used to treat an enlarged prostate. Finasteride not only lowers DHT levels in the prostate and blood but also decreases DHT levels in the scalp, which should improve the growth phase of hair. While 5 mg of finasteride is used to treat BPH, a lower dose of 1 mg suffices for male-pattern baldness. This 1-mg dose of finasteride, called Propecia®, must be taken for six to 12 months before you can tell whether it's working.

Though there are few side effects with Propecia®, the ones that tend to get a guy's attention are lower sexual drive, or libido, problems with erections, and smaller amounts of ejaculate. Most men have none of these problems. Like topical minoxidil, Propecia® must be taken for the long term to maintain results. If Propecia® provides hair growth or prevents hair loss in a man, and he stops the medication, his loss will accelerate and his hair will return to the baseline as if the medication had never been used. Studies are underway currently to find out whether taking both minoxidil and Propecia® works better than taking either medication alone.

Several surgical procedures are used to treat male-pattern baldness. Hair plugs can be taken from areas with a lot of hair, like the back of the head, and moved to areas where hair is sparse. Transplanted hairs follow the growth patterns of the areas from which they came, not the ones to which they were transplanted. In other words, they do not shed, and baldness does not recur. Hair plugs may be as big as half a centimeter or as small as a single hair. The smaller the plugs, the less noticeable and more dispersed and natural the end result. Micrografts (grafts with 1 to 2 hairs) and mini-grafts (grafts with 3 to 4 hairs) when used in large numbers (1,000 to 2,000 grafts) are often quite effective. It may take one or two sessions for a natural looking result. Each session lasts four to six hours. The smaller the plugs and the greater the number of plugs, the more expensive the hair transplantation. Smaller plugs cost more because more transplants and more sessions usually are involved. After transplantation, hair follicles usually go into an extended resting (telogen) phase of three to six months before beginning to grow again.

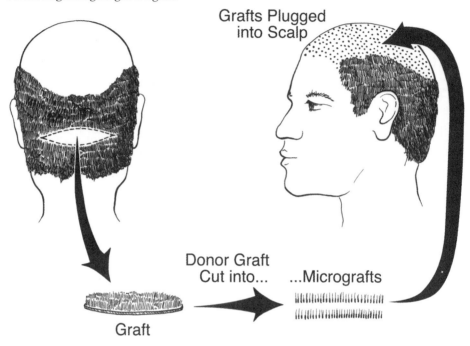

Hair plugs are taken from areas of good hair growth and moved to areas of baldness: a redistribution of hair.

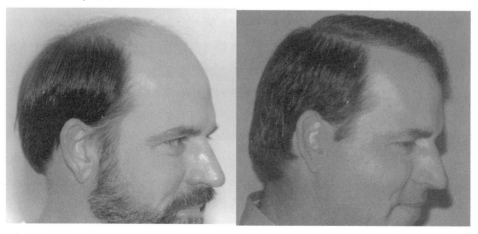

(Left) Patient with typical male pattern baldness. (Right) After a micrograft session. (Photograph kindly supplied by Dr. Alfonso Barrera. Houston, Texas.)

Another surgical treatment for baldness is *scalp reduction*. This is an excision or removal of bare parts of the scalp to reduce the size of the bald area. The scalp is then sutured together. A third treatment is the transfer of flaps of scalp that contain hair to areas that don't. The pieces of scalp are called temporoparietal and occipital (TPO) flaps. This surgery often takes several stages to complete. A final technique is to implant tissue expanders that expand the hair-bearing parts of the scalp. Afterwards, scalp reduction of the bald areas is done. The hair-bearing part of the scalp that is expanded is then used to cover the bald part of the scalp that has been cut out. Because the tissue is expanded, the closure is without tension and gives a better cosmetic result. Transplantation of plugs can be added later for the best cosmetic results. All of these surgical procedures are done under local anesthesia on an outpatient basis.

Artificial hair is also an option. Implanting artificial hair, however, is not recommended. Artificial fibers often cause local allergy-like reactions; they also carry an increased chance of infection and scarring. Weaving or braiding artificial or real hair into existing hair is an alternative to implantation. Weaving, sometimes called a "hair system," must be adjusted in a styling session every month or so. Finally, toupees, some of which can be virtually imperceptible (except to the wallet), may be glued to the scalp or clipped onto existing hair.

Patchy Hair Loss

Alopecia areata, or hair loss in small, circumscribed areas of the scalp, can occur suddenly. Sometimes all the body hair falls out, but usually the scalp is not red or scaly. The cause of this patchy hair loss, in general, is not known. Hair growth normally recurs, but it can take several months. Because inflammation and the immune system likely are involved in alopecia areata, steroids may improve the condition.

Patchy hair loss may also occur with a red and scaly scalp. This may be caused by a bacterial or fungal infection. Plucking the hair to look for spores that indicate fungal infection or head lice, or culturing the hair will often result in diagnosis. If fungal or bacterial infection is the cause, oral or topical medications and shampoos are the treatment of choice.

Diffuse Hair Loss

Diffuse alopecia, or hair loss, may occur over a period of weeks or months. Some particular event, occurring within three months of onset, usually precipitates the condition. This may include the use of medications such as heparin, Coumadin®, amphetamines, some antihypertensive medications, and others. Chemotherapy for treating cancer may also cause diffuse hair loss. Chemotherapy usually is harmful to hair during its growth phase. Since around 90 percent of all hair follicles are in the growth phase at any given time, chemotherapeutic agents may cause a dramatic hair loss. Often hair regrowth occurs when treatment is concluded.

Other causes of sudden hair loss include traumatic events such as surgery, crash diets, and severe illness. General debilitation from systemic illness or nutritional disorders may also cause hair loss. Finally, hormone disorders such as too little thyroid hormone (hypothyroidism) or too much thyroid hormone (hyperthyroidism) can cause hair loss.

Diffuse hair loss is sometimes associated with an inflamed or scaly scalp such as occurs with psoriasis or seborrheic dermatitis. Rarely do these conditions in themselves cause hair loss, but scratching can exacerbate the loss. The treatment of these disorders depends on the particular cause. Any specific nutritional disorder or systemic disease resulting in hair loss should be treated as well.

The Bottom Line

- The most common type of baldness is male-pattern baldness. Genes and hormones cause this.

- Many men are comfortable with their baldness, and no therapy is recommended.

- Medical therapy is available for male-pattern baldness. The authors (and the sons of the bald one) plan to keep abreast of promising new treatments.

- Surgical therapy is possible and the results can look good, but it is expensive.

- If you have concerns regarding hair loss or you have hair loss associated with a red and scaly scalp, see your primary care physician or a dermatologist.

13

Male Menopause
It's not just for women anymore

Is male menopause just a cute idea to help explain a guy's midlife crisis, is it a ploy to get a little sympathy from women, or does it really exist? The medical definition of menopause is cessation of menses, which implies that a woman can no longer have children. Men do not have menstrual cycles, which is one good reason why they will never get much sympathy from females on this menopause issue. And there is no maximum age for a man to conceive a child; even men in their nineties have conceived children. So, in a strict sense, male menopause doesn't exist.

Nevertheless, some men in their forties, fifties, and sixties experience problems with erections, decreased sexual drive or libido, hot flashes, depression, mood swings, irritability, weakness, lethargy, and loss of calcium in bone. These are similar to the symptoms women have when they undergo menopause. So, if we use a looser definition, some men do indeed experience menopause.

What are some of the changes happening to men as they age? One significant change is that testosterone levels tend to decrease. Not only are testosterone levels lower, but the normal biorhythm of testosterone levels—high in the morning and low in the afternoon—may be lost. Testosterone levels in the bloodstream tend to be the same throughout the day in older men. This finding is a clue as to why men may undergo menopause. Remember, testosterone is one of the major male hormones made in the testicles. It is necessary for making sperm, maintaining high sexual drive (libido), growing facial hair, and developing that baritone voice.

Young men with low testosterone are said to have *hypogonadism:* They have problems with making sperm and may not be interested in sex. They also may have loss of muscle, loss of calcium in their bones (osteoporosis), lethargy, and depression.

Does this sound familiar? These symptoms of low testosterone are the same ones associated with male menopause. That's why many people think men have male menopause because their testosterone levels are too low. It's also why some people think men who have signs of male menopause can be treated with testosterone.

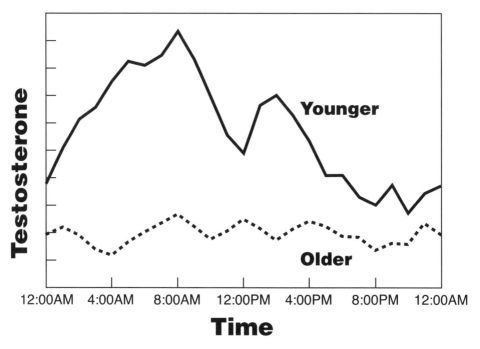

Younger men get a surge of testosterone in the morning that recedes in the late afternoon and evening. Older men do not have this biorhythm and tend to have lower levels of testosterone.

Men do have some decline in reproductive function as they get older; it's just not as profound as in women. Sperm counts usually don't change much. Instead, sperm movement, or motility, tends to decrease as men age. The sperm just don't have that get-up-and-go anymore. There is also some scarring and other changes going on in the testicle. But overall, there are few dramatic changes to sperm in men hitting their twilight years. Remember this if you are older and considering unprotected intercourse with a woman who is not menopausal. Do you really want a baby when you are 90? Getting old is not a good method of birth control for men.

As discussed in chapter 8, changes in erections, ability to ejaculate, and sexual drive occur as a man gets older. We are not talking about changes at age 90, but ones that occur in the twenties and thirties. A 35-year-old came to our office with concerns about his ability to have sex. He thought he had an unusual and significant problem that needed fixing. Previously, he had been able to have sex four times a night. But over the past couple of years he could have sex and ejaculate only once or twice each night. We assured him that this is normal as men get older, and he left the office cured.

It's hard to have a lot of sympathy for a guy who can have intercourse only twice in one evening. Yet most men are not aware that their sexuality changes as they get older. For example, ejaculation is different in a guy of 30 from what it was when he first ejaculated. His first ejaculate could hit the ceiling, but at age 30 he can barely get it off the ground. The table below shows some of the effects of aging on sexuality. As you can see, it's not all downhill as a man ages; it's just different. One aspect of sex, having more control over ejaculations, tends to get better with age.

Changes in Male Sexuality with Aging

Function	Effect
Arousal	Decreased
Sense of impending orgasm	Decreased
Force of ejaculation	Decreased
Contractions of perineal muscles with ejaculation	Decreased
Testicular elevation	Testes hang lower
Refractory period (time before one can ejaculate again)	Longer
Loss of erection after ejaculation	Quicker
Ejaculatory control	Increased

Changes in sexuality depend on the individual and vary considerably. One man may have a more significant decrease in sexual drive than another. Furthermore, one man's experience may vary from setting to setting or from day to day. For example, under normal circumstances a guy may not care much about sex. When he does have intercourse, he may do it only once on any one day. Take that same guy, put him in Hawaii, and he may turn into a sexual beast able to have sex four or five times a night. Finally, other contributing factors such as illness, medications, loss of a partner, or a partner's waning interest in sex can affect a man's sexual drive as well as his ability to get an erection.

Testosterone has little to do with a man's erections. Yet many men seek androgens, such as testosterone, to boost their sexual prowess. Taking testosterone may help men who have mild problems with erections. And as discussed earlier, it often helps improve sexual drive in men with low testosterone levels. But it rarely does anything for men who have significant problems with erections. For these men, a pill (such as Viagra®), use of a vacuum constriction device, injection therapy, or a penile prosthesis is usually more effective.

Like women, men tend to lose muscle mass and strength, gain body fat, and develop osteoporosis as they get older. The loss of bone makes a man more susceptible to hip and other bone fractures. Low testosterone levels in a young man will cause the same problems, and testosterone supplementation will reverse the process. Therefore, giving extra testosterone to older men with low testosterone levels may result in an increase in muscle mass and strength, a loss of body fat, and an increase in bone calcium.

Who Should Get Testosterone Supplementation?

There are probably many women out there who think that no man should receive extra testosterone. As men get older, their testosterone levels decrease, and they finally become more tranquil. Why reverse that process? So they can feel and act like Rocky Balboa? These feelings are understandable, but there are legitimate reasons for a man taking testosterone, and some men want to be like Rocky their whole lives. Current research suggests that testosterone therapy is likely to help certain men, and it might benefit others, but it does not help everyone.

A man with low testosterone and a low sexual drive is a great candidate for testosterone therapy. If a guy's testosterone is low, and he has a mild problem with impotency, extra testosterone may improve erections. A middle-aged or older man with low testosterone who is suffering from osteoporosis, mood swings, or loss of a sense of well-being may benefit from testosterone. Finally, if a man has normal levels of testosterone, he will not benefit from extra testosterone.

A man's testosterone levels may be low for reasons other than male menopause. Trauma to the testicles, undescended testicles as a child, other hormonal problems such as thyroid or pituitary problems, mumps that have affected the testicles, radiation therapy or chemotherapy, some medications, and certain genetic and congenital problems can cause lower testosterone level. If these problems occur before a male reaches puberty, they may cause delayed puberty. If any of these problems decrease testosterone after puberty, the same symptoms affecting men with male menopause can occur. Therefore, for a variety of reasons, some young men with low testosterone levels may also benefit from testosterone therapy.

The Dark Side of Testosterone

We are not talking here about the possibility of turning a perfect gentleman into a beer-swigging, belching animal, but about the effects testosterone can have on the prostate, on blood levels, and on other aspects of physical health.

As stated earlier, prostate cancer is the most commonly diagnosed cancer in men in the United States, and testosterone supports its growth. Consequently, the possibility that testosterone therapy may cause prostate cancer is a concern, though no current evidence supports this. But if a man has prostate cancer when starting testosterone or happens to develop prostate cancer while he is on this therapy, the testosterone probably will make the prostate cancer grow faster. Testosterone also may cause prostate tissue to grow or swell and cause some of the obstructive symptoms of prostatism or BPH. So any man with prostate problems probably should not take testosterone, and all men on testosterone should be followed closely with PSA levels and rectal examinations in case prostate cancer develops.

Testosterone can increase the number of red blood cells so that the blood becomes heavier and thicker than it should be. Though highly unlikely, this could cause a stroke. Men on testosterone should have their blood levels (hemoglobin or hematocrit) checked to make sure they are not "overtanked with blood." Testosterone can also cause sleep apnea—temporarily ceasing to breathe when asleep. A man with sleep apnea may have a restless night, snore, or feel tired in the morning. If you have or develop sleep apnea while on testosterone, alert your physician. Bigger breasts or *gynecomastia*, weight gain from fluid retention or increased muscle mass, and cardiovascular or liver problems, though unlikely, may also occur with testosterone therapy.

How to Get That Testosterone Boost

Shots, patches, or a lotion are currently the best way to get those testosterone levels up to normal. Testosterone pills are also available, but most of them have the potential to cause serious liver disease. There is an oral testosterone that is *not* harmful to the liver; its generic name is testosterone undecanoate. Testosterone undecanoate is available in Europe but not in the United States. So be careful about taking testosterone pills if you live in the U.S.

Even if access is not a problem, the testosterone undecanoate pill has its disadvantages. First, it should be taken three times a day. Many women don't remember to take their birth control pills once a day; what are the odds a man will remember three times a day? In addition, testosterone pills do not give the natural peaks in the morning and low levels in the afternoon and evening. Finally, they can cause gastrointestinal problems.

Okay, so what is a good, available way to get testosterone? Let's set expectations straight from the beginning. Right now there is no perfect method of testosterone supplementation. One method that has been around for a long time is testosterone shots. These are given in the muscle of the buttocks or thigh once every two to four weeks, usually in the doctor's office. Yes, it hurts, but not too bad. Probably the biggest drawback to shots is the nuisance of frequent visits to the doctor's office. An alternative is asking the man's partner to learn to give the shots; in fact, the partner may enjoy it. Finally, the shots can cause a big peak of testosterone (more than is natural) that drops to subnormal levels before the next shot is due. These "big highs" and "low lows" can be stressful.

Patches are another source of testosterone. These are placed on the skin on a daily basis. Their advantage is that they are not shots, a man can apply them himself, and they provide a natural peak in the morning and a low later in the day. One patch, Androderm® (made by SmithKline), is relatively expensive and can irritate the skin, but a man can place it on many parts of the body, like the back, stomach, arms, and legs. This is in contrast to another patch, called Testoderm® (made by Alza), which is put on the scrotum. The advantage of the scrotum patch is that it allows slightly more testosterone to be absorbed and is less likely to irritate the skin than the body patch. The scrotum patch will stick better if the scrotum is shaved. This is different from shaving your face, but most guys are pros at shaving and will not shave too aggressively down there. Alza has subsequently come out with a body patch as well.

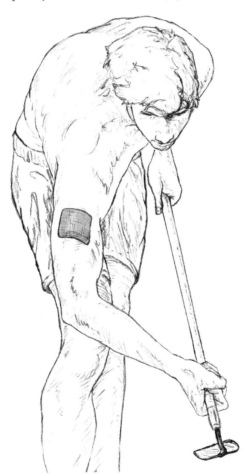

A man wearing a testosterone patch on his arm.

Potential methods for getting that testosterone boost in the future include a pill that you put under your tongue, airpowered shots without needles, creams and lotions that contain testosterone (one of which, AndroGel® 1%, just received FDA approval and is now available), and better patches. These will be welcome additions. Still, finding a perfect way to deliver testosterone is like finding a car that will be perfect for everyone. It's nice to have some choices, but each man must decide for himself. If you don't like one method, try another.

Every Man's Guide to Testosterone

Here are the fundamentals for guys who want to be on testosterone. First of all, make sure you have a good reason. At this time the primary indication for testosterone therapy is a low testosterone level and low libido. As we learn more about the beneficial effects and problems of testosterone therapy, the indications may well change.

A man should be aware that testosterone therapy likely will affect his fertility. As discussed in chapter 5, on infertility, a high level of testosterone in the testicle is necessary for sperm production. When a man receives extra testosterone by shot, patch, or lotion, the testosterone signals his pituitary gland that he has "enough." The pituitary then shuts off its signal—luteinizing hormone or LH—to the testicle, and the testicle shuts off its production of testosterone. So even though the testosterone levels in the bloodstream are normal, the levels in the testicles are low, and this shuts off the production of sperm. If testosterone therapy stops, the testicle usually, but not always, recovers. Therefore, if a man wants to have kids later, he should not take testosterone.

There may be ways to increase testosterone levels without hurting sperm production. One method is to take other hormones (clomiphene citrate or human chorionic gonadotropin) to stimulate the testicle to make more testosterone. If a man is young and wants to have kids but has low testosterone, he should discuss this issue with his physician.

Finally, as discussed, testosterone therapy may affect a man's prostate or breasts, and it can cause sleep apnea. If a man has prostate or breast cancer (yes, men can have breast cancer, though it is rare), severe BPH, or sleep apnea, he should not start testosterone therapy. A physician should get a good history, check the prostate by rectal examination, and draw a PSA level to make sure there is no evidence of prostate cancer before prescribing testosterone. A man should discuss with his doctor the pros and cons of testosterone therapy and all the potential side effects before taking it.

Once a man starts testosterone therapy, he should make sure his physician follows up with him. After three or four months of treatment, the doctor should check his testosterone levels with a blood test. The doctor should also check the red-blood-cell level (draw a hematocrit or hemoglobin) and the PSA level. If the testosterone level is normal with treatment but is not giving the desired effect, stop the therapy. Then, with a physician, reevaluate for other medical or psychological problems that may cause the adverse symptoms and consider other medical treatments or mental health counseling.

Last but not least, a man on testosterone should have frequent rectal examinations to make sure no prostate cancer has developed. As far as we are concerned, a man on testosterone can't have too many rectal examinations. In fact, any man on testosterone should probably see his physician every six to twelve months for an interview, rectal exam, and PSA level. Even this may not catch every problem, but it is a thorough approach to keeping your health while on testosterone.

The Bottom Line

- In a strict sense, there is no such thing as male menopause. Most men maintain the ability to conceive children as they age, even into their nineties.

- Many men experience some of the same symptoms as women who are going through menopause: loss of sexual drive, hot flashes, loss of vigor, depression, osteoporosis, and so forth. Thus, in a loose sense, male menopause does exist.

- Testosterone tends to decrease as men age.

- Some symptoms of male menopause, in particular low libido, may be due to lower testosterone levels.

- The current indications for testosterone therapy are a low level of testosterone and low libido. Other symptoms, such as a decreased sense of well-being, mild erectile dysfunction, and osteoporosis may indicate—in the presence of low testosterone levels—testosterone therapy.

- If a man has a history of prostate cancer, breast cancer, severe prostatism or BPH, sleep apnea, or is trying to conceive, he should not take testosterone.

- Currently, the best way to get extra testosterone is by patches, shots, or lotion. A testosterone pill that dissolves under the tongue may be available soon.

- Men on testosterone should see their physicians every six to twelve months for an interview, a rectal examination, and a PSA level.

14

General Health

Healthy body for healthy sperm, erections, prostate . . .

This is a book about men's health; it is about issues specific to men, like impotency and prostate disease. We have purposefully stayed away from general health concerns, such as heart disease, since having a heart is not unique to men. But a chapter on overall health is worthwhile: if a man's body is not generally healthy, his testicles, penis, and prostate won't be either. To keep sperm happy and the penis up, cultivate good health habits. Most of these are just common sense, but we could all use a little reminder of what to do and what not to do.

The foremost health rule is "Don't do drugs." The definition of drugs can be quite broad. Coffee? Cigarettes and alcohol? These deserve their own categories. But we're talking here about street drugs. Lots of guys have done them. What is past is past, but do not take them again.

If a man has not taken any street drugs in the past, he should not start now. It's just not worth it. For one thing, many of these drugs are truly addicting, even with one use. Cocaine, for example, sounds great, but some people have become addicted—and ruined their lives—after trying it once. Have you heard of Len Bias? The guy was on top of the world. He was a great basketball player out of Maryland and the first draft pick for the NBA. A night of celebrating with cocaine left him dead. Well, those things always happen to somebody else, but if you take these drugs, it could be you.

Even marijuana can be bad. For one thing, it's hard to concentrate when you are high from smoking a joint. When that happens, it's harder to drive, to focus on your studies, to work at a job, and to talk to people coherently. Marijuana also lowers testosterone levels. This can drastically reduce sperm counts and decrease sexual drive enough to cause difficulty with having sex. We just had a patient who was trying to have a baby, but his sperm counts were too low. He smoked marijuana, and we advised him to quit. Four months later his sperm counts were still low. Upon questioning, he said he was still smoking marijuana and acted surprised, as if he had never been told that it could harm both his sperm and his testicles. He may have been so high the first time that he forgot. When a man quits smoking marijuana, the testicles usually get better, but it takes time.

Excessive alcohol is bad for the liver, testicles, and brain. The calories from alcohol contribute to obesity. One or two glasses of wine or a couple of drinks a day are not bad for you. In fact, researchers believe this amount of alcohol increases the good cholesterol—HDL-cholesterol—that helps prevent heart disease. But the fact that just because one or two glasses of wine or a couple of drinks may be okay doesn't mean three or four are better. They're not. And just because one or two drinks a day are all right does not mean that you can save it all up and have 14 glasses on Friday night. That's bad for the brain and testicles.

Now let's take a look at tobacco—and not just cigarettes. Cigars are "in" with celebrities, like Arnold Schwarzenegger, who appear with cigars on the covers of magazines. This encourages millions of men and women to go to cigar dens. Then there is chewing tobacco. Tobacco is bad for you, no matter the form. In addition to causing lung cancer, strokes, and heart attacks, chewing tobacco and smoking can harm sperm production and make it harder to conceive.

Smoking can also make it more difficult for a man to get it up. If he cannot conceive and cannot have intercourse, well, can he at least smoke and kiss? No. Smoking and chewing tobacco can cause mouth and throat cancer, which could result in the removal of half a man's face just to save his life. That would definitely hurt kissing. With nicotine gum, nicotine patches, Zyban® and smoking clinics available, there are plenty of ways to help men quit smoking or chewing. The man who quits, will live longer and better.

Some folks consider coffee a drug. Coffee does have some stimulating effects, but that is not all bad. As with many things in life, moderation is good. To avoid an upset stomach or too great an increase in heart rate, limit coffee intake to about two cups a day. For people who do not drink coffee at all, that's okay, you can still be cool.

No drugs, no excess alcohol, no smoking. What can a guy do? He can eat well. That does not mean he should eat a lot, but that he should eat the right food. We can't get into everything that is good and bad for you here. Just read some of the hundreds of books on nutrition, foods, and dieting.

Though diets and recommendations come and go, some advice has withstood the test of time. For example, avoid adding salt to your food. Most food already has enough salt, and too much can increase blood pressure. You can't help eating some fat, but try not to eat saturated fats, such as in deep-fried foods, hard margarine, pastries, and cookies. Fiber may not taste good, but your heart likes it. Fiber from grains, vegetables, and fruits lowers cholesterol levels. Vitamins from fruits and vegetables or from a multivitamin with antioxidants, such as vitamins C, E, and beta-carotene, may keep cholesterol from blocking your arteries and prevent cancer.

Staying healthy without exercise is difficult. A man doesn't have to do a lot, but some extra activity is good for the body. Exercising at least three times a week for a minimum of 20 minutes is good. Thirty minutes is better. Getting the heart going and putting in some effort is better than non-aerobic exercise. But any exercise, even a brisk walk after dinner, is good.

Be smart when starting to exercise after living a sedentary lifestyle. A sister-in-law challenged one of us (J.P.) to a five-mile race. To meet the challenge, he started an aggressive running program on the treadmill. Bad, bad, bad. A severe, exercise-induced bursitis in his knee left him virtually unable to walk or do any other fun activities. Be smarter than that. Start slowly; then increase endurance, speed, or weights. Get a trainer, doctor, or experienced friend to help develop a healthy exercise plan so that you avoid injury or heart attack. Do exercises you enjoy. If you do, you're more likely to continue exercising, and that's the way to stay healthy.

One health tip many people do not think about is "Everything in moderation." Obviously, drinking too much alcohol is bad for you. So if you drink, do so in moderation. But virtually anything can be done to an extreme. People have even drowned from drinking too much water. Some women who exercise to an extreme amount may have irregular periods. Presumably, men who exercise to an extreme also may have subtle hormonal problems that can affect fertility or sex drive. (We're talking about those who run ultramarathons or spend six hours daily in the gym. You know who you are.) So when drinking coffee, exercising, working, sleeping, or having some beer, do it in moderation.

All sorts of other suggestions are worth a mention. Get a reasonable amount of sleep, see a physician for routine checkups, and learn to deal with stress. Men who work with solvents, oils, pesticides, herbicides, and other poisons should be aware that these can be absorbed through the skin or inhaled. They have the potential to affect many organs in the body, including the testicles, where young sperm are developing. If you have to work with toxins, minimize your contact by using them in well-ventilated areas, by wearing protective clothing, and if you get them on your skin, by washing the area as soon as possible. Finally, taking a baby aspirin every day, or one aspirin every other day, may help prevent heart attacks.

Some Concluding Thoughts

We are undoubtedly leaving out other healthy habits. The best habit of all may be to keep up with the latest research on how to live healthy. Some suggestions from the research will be a flash in the pan, but generally they are not harmful.

We admit that following these good habits is no guarantee. One of our mother-in-laws ate vegetables her whole life, and got plenty of beta-carotenes, but still developed breast cancer. Life is not fair. But without those vegetables and her other healthy habits, the cancer may have been worse or developed earlier. The man with healthy habits, even if he is infertile, impotent, or develops prostate cancer, will stay healthier and enjoy life longer. A little effort now will help you live a fuller and richer life. Have fun.

The Bottom Line

- Don't do drugs. Don't even smoke marijuana; it lowers testosterone levels.

- Do not smoke cigarettes, cigars, or pipes. Smoking not only affects the lungs but also is bad for sperm and erections. And don't chew tobacco. It also affects sperm, and it may cause mouth cancer.

- If you drink alcohol, do so in moderation.

- Eat healthy by eating a variety of foods. Watch your saturated fat intake and eat plenty of vegetables, fruits, breads, and pastas.

- Exercise at least three times a week.

- Be moderate in all you do. Your body likes moderation.

Appendix 1
Support Groups & Resources

IMPOTENCE

American Diabetes Association, Inc.
1660 Duke Street
Alexandria, VA 22314
1-800-232-3472

Provides information on professional meetings, subscriptions, membership, and general information about diabetes.

American Foundation for Urological Disease, Inc. (AFUD)
300 West Pratt Street, Suite 401
Baltimore, MD 21201
1-800-242-2383

Impotence Anonymous and I-ANON Chapters
1-800-669-1603

Provides a list of urologists with the latest treatment options for impotency and lists of local support groups.

Impotence World Association (IWA)
10400 Little Patuxent Parkway, Suite 485
Columbia, MD 21044-3502

Send three dollars to the above address with a request for educational materials or referral lists of local physicians and therapists who treat impotency.

Osbon Foundation
1-800-433-4215

Provides basic information on impotency.

Retired Persons Services, Inc.
Provider of the AARP Pharmacy Service.
1-800-289-6031

SIECUS, The Sexuality Information and Education Council of the United States
130 West 42nd Street, Suite 350
New York, NY 10036
1-212-819-9770

Refers callers to specialists and provides information on sex education for children.

INCONTINENCE

NAFC (National Association for Continence)
1-800-80-US-TOO

Provides a quarterly newsletter and information on local support groups and prostate cancer (see US TOO under prostate cancer resources).

INFERTILITY

American Society for Reproductive Medicine
1-205-978-5000

Provides educational materials relating to infertility.

Resolve
1310 Broadway
Somerville, MA 02144-1744
Business Office 1-617-623-1156
Helpline 1-617-623-0744

Provides listings of local support groups and educational materials on infertility and adoption.

PROSTATE CANCER

American Cancer Society
1-800-ACS-2345 (1-800-227-2345)

Provides pamphlets on prostate cancer.

The National Cancer Institute's Cancer Information Service (CIS)
1-800-4-CANCER (1-800-422-6237)
In Hawaii on Oahu, call 514-1234; from other islands call collect.

Provides publications on cancer and specialists to speak with callers.

Prostate Health Council of the American Foundation of Urologic Disease
300 West Pratt Street, Suite 401
Baltimore, MD 21201
1-800-242-2383

US TOO International, Inc.
1-800-808-7866

Provides quarterly newsletters and information on local support groups.

SEX THERAPY

American Association of Sex Educators, Counselors, and Therapists
435 N. Michigan Avenue
Chicago, IL 60611
1-312-644-0828

Gives referrals to qualified sex therapists in your region.

SIECUS, The Sexuality Information and Education Council of the U.S.
1-212-819-9770

Has a database of information related to sexual problems.

TESTICULAR CANCER

American Cancer Society
1-800-ACS-2345

Provides pamphlets and information on testicular cancer and how to perform testicular self-examination.

Appendix 2
Pharmaceuticals & Medical Devices

MEDICATION or DEVICE	MANUFACTURER	PHONE NUMBER/WEB SITES	TREATMENT
Androderm®	SmithKline	1-800-454-2436 www.testosteronesource.com	testosterone replacement
AndroGel®	UNIMED	www.androgel.com	testosterone replacement
Cardura®	Pfizer	1-800-438-1985 www.pfizer.com	BPH medication
Casodex®	AstraZeneca	1-800-237-8898 www.casodex.com	prostate cancer medication
Caverject®	Pharmacia Upjohn	1-800-867-7042 www.caverject.com	erectile dysfunction medication
Dura II Prosthesis®	Timm Medical	1-800-344-9688 www.timmmedical.com	penile prosthesis
Dynaflex Prosthesis®	AMS	1-800-843-4315 www.visitAMS.com	penile prosthesis
Edex®	Schwartz Pharma	1-800-558-5114 www.edex.com	erectile dysfunction medication
Eulexin®	Schering Laboratories	1-800-521-7157 www.prostatecancer.com	prostate cancer medication
Flomax®	Boehringer Ingelheim	1-800-796-3649 www.flomax-bph.com	BPH medication
Hytrin®	Abbott Laboratories	1-800-222-6885 www.hytrin.com	BPH medication
Indigo®	Johnson & Johnson	1-888-9INDIGO www.indigomedical.com	laser treatment for BPH
Lupron®	TAP	1-800-621-1020 www.tapurology.com	prostate cancer medication
Mark II Prosthesis®	Mentor	1-800-221-5517 www.mentorcorp.com	penile prosthesis
MUSE®	Vivus	1-888-367-MUSE www.vivus.com	erectile dysfunction medication
Nilandron®	Hoechst-Marion Roussel	1-800-362-7466 www.aventis.com	prostate cancer medication

MEDICATION or DEVICE	MANUFACTURER	PHONE NUMBER/WEB SITES	TREATMENT
Propecia®	Merck www.propecia.com	1-800-830-7375	hair replacement medication
Proscar®	Merck	1-800-830-7375 www.proscar.com	BPH medication
Prostatron®	EDAP Technomed	1-800-933-TUMT www.edaptechnomed.com	microwave treatment (TUMT) for BPH
Proxeed®	Sigma-Tau	1-877-Proxeed www.proxeed.com	natural supplement for the treatment of male infertility
Rejoyn®	Gain	1-651-659-2407 www.rejoyn.com	treatment for erectile dysfunction
Rigiscan®	Timm	1-800-344-9688 www.timmmedical.com	a computer to measure nighttime erections
Targis®	Urologix	1-888-229-0772 www.targis.com	microwave treatment (TUMT) for BPH
Testoderm®	Alza	1-800-634-8977 www.alza.com	testosterone replacement
VTS PROVu™	VidaMed	1-800-879-5070 www.vidamed.com	radiofrequency (TUNA) for BPH treatment
Ultrex Prosthesis®	AMS	1-800-843-4315 www.visitAMS.com	penile prosthesis
Uprima®	TAP	1-800-621-1020 www.tapurology.com	medication for treatment of erectile dysfunction
Viagra®	Pfizer	1-888-4VIAGRA www.viagra.com	erectile dysfunction medication
Zoladex®	AstraZeneca	1-800-237-8898 www.prostateinfo.com	prostate cancer medication
Zyban®	GlaxoWellcome	1-800-822-7848 www.zyban.com	medication to help quit smoking

Appendix 3
Glossary

Abscess - An infection that turns into pus and becomes walled off and isolated. Because an abscess is walled off, treating it with antibiotics is difficult. Usually it must be drained with a needle or by surgery.

Alopecia areata - A patchy loss of hair from the scalp or other part of the body such as the beard or eyebrows. The loss of hair occurs without redness or any signs of inflammation.

Anagen - Growing phase of hair.

Anastomosis - The connection of two tubes, such as in the reanastomosis of the vas deferens during vasectomy reversal.

Anejaculation - Inability to ejaculate. This is common in men with spinal cord injuries.

Antiandrogen - A medication that blocks the effects of testosterone or other androgens. Antiandrogens are often used to treat prostate cancer that has spread.

Arteriography - X-ray test in which contrast (dye) is injected into arteries to see whether they are blocked.

Atrophic - Shrinking, such as in atrophy of the testicles.

Azoospermia - Absence of sperm in the ejaculate.

BPH (benign prostatic hyperplasia) - A growth of tissue within the prostate that blocks the urethra and makes urination difficult.

Balanitis - Infection of the head (glans) of the penis.

Biopsy gun - Device that uses a spring to push a needle into the prostate so quickly that a sample of tissue may be obtained without pain. Transrectal ultrasound guides the needle into the correct area of the prostate.

Bone scan - X-ray test that shows whether cancer has spread to bone. A small amount of radioactive material injected into the patient concentrates in bone where there is a lot of activity such as cancer, an old fracture, or arthritis. It can show whether prostate cancer has spread to bone.

Caput - Beginning or head of the epididymis.

Cauda - Tail or end of the epididymis. The cauda epididymis is connected to the vas deferens.

Cavernosometry - A test in which fluid is injected into the penis and pressure within the penis is measured to determine whether venous leak is causing impotency. Men with venous leak show low pressures.

Clomiphene citrate - A medication that stimulates the testicle to make testosterone. It is sometimes used to try to increase sperm counts in men or to stimulate ovulation in women.

Corpora - The erectile chambers of the penis.

Cryptorchidism - An undescended testicle.

Cystoscopy - Inspection of the bladder with a telescope.

Detumesced - Flaccid, as when an erection goes down.

Duplex ultrasound - An ultrasound that examines the arteries of the penis. It helps determine whether a man has impotency from disease of the arteries.

Ejaculation - Fluid and sperm "coming" out of the penis during sex, masturbation, and wet dreams.

Embolization - To block a blood vessel. It is a treatment for varicoceles performed by radiologists.

Empirical therapy - The use of unproven medications or treatment. Empirical treatments may or may not help.

Epididymal aspiration - Sucking up sperm from the epididymis. The sperm is injected into an egg as part of in vitro fertilization (IVF). Epididymal aspiration, for example, is useful for men without a vas deferens who want to conceive.

Epididymal blowout - Rupture of the epididymis because of increased pressure in a man who has had a vasectomy. While painless, it causes a blockage within the epididymis.

Epididymis - Coiled tube behind the testicle that transports sperm from the testicle to the vas deferens, stores sperm, and helps sperm to mature and becomes capable of fertilizing an egg.

Epididymitis - Infection of the epididymis.

Epididymo-orchitis - Infection of the epididymis and testicle.

FSH (follicle stimulating hormone) - A hormone made by the pituitary that stimulates the testicle to make sperm. A high level of FSH means the testicles are not functioning well.

Fractured penis - Occurs when the lining of the erectile bodies (tunica albuginea) tears from the bending of an erect penis. A fractured penis is swollen and painful.

Frequency - Frequent urination. This is common in men with BPH.

GnRH - Hormone produced by the hypothalamus in the brain. It stimulates the pituitary gland to release FSH and LH, which in turn stimulates the testicles.

GnRH analog - A medication that acts like GnRH. When given in pulses, a GnRH analog stimulates the pituitary to release FSH and LH. But given at a constant dose, the GnRH analog decreases the pituitary hormones FSH and LH. This lowers testosterone and is a treatment for men with prostate cancer that has spread.

Germ cells - Developing sperm (and eggs).

Glans penis - Head of the penis.

Gross hematuria - Blood visible in urine. This can be a sign of cancer and means you should see a urologist.

Gynecomastia - Enlargement of the male breasts.

Hematocrit - A hemoglobin or blood level.

Hematospermia - Blood in the ejaculate.

Hematuria - Blood in the urine. Hematuria can be gross (visible) or microscopic (detected on a urinalysis).

Hormones - A chemical made in one part of the body that gets into the blood and affects an organ somewhere else. FSH, LH, and testosterone are examples of hormones.

Hydrocele - Fluid around the testicle. Large hydroceles make the scrotum look big.

Hyperprolactinemia - High prolactin levels in the blood. Hyperprolactinemia can result from a tumor in the pituitary and can cause infertility as well as impotency.

Hyperthyriodism - Elevated thyroid levels. This may affect fertility and cause other health problems.

Hypogonadism - Literally, small testicles. But most physicians use this term for testicles that are not working well (making low amounts of sperm and testosterone).

Hypospadias - Condition in which the opening of the urethra, where urine and semen come out, is not at the end of the penis but closer to the body on the underside of the penis. This can be corrected with surgery.

Hypothyroidism - Low thyroid levels. This may affect fertility.

Idiopathic infertility - Infertility from an unknown cause.

Incontinence - Uncontrolled leakage of urine.

Inguinal - The upper thigh or groin area. This is where a hernia operation is often performed.

Intravenous pyelogram - X-ray test to examine the kidneys, ureters, and bladder. Contrast (dye) is injected into the veins which concentrates in the kidneys and allows these organs to be seen by x-rays.

Krueger's strict criteria - A different, more picky method of assessing sperm shape. This is part of a semen analysis.

LH (luteinizing hormones) - A hormone made by the pituitary gland that stimulates Leydig cells in the testicle to make testosterone.

Leydig cells - Cells in the testicle that make testosterone.

Libido - Sexual drive or horniness.

Lymph nodes - Small pieces of tissue, about the size of a dime, that lymph (fluid and white blood cells) goes through. Big lymph nodes may mean that a cancer or infection is going through them.

Morphology - The part of a semen analysis that assesses the shape of sperm. Abnormal-shaped sperm probably do not fertilize the egg well (this does not mean that abnormal children will result).

Motility - The percentage of sperm that are moving.

Nocturia - Urinating at night. Often a sign of benign prostatic hyperplasia (BPH).

Nocturnal penile tumescence - Erections in the middle of the night. Nighttime erections are normal. If a person complains of impotency but has normal nocturnal erections, the impotency may be caused by psychological problems or anxiety.

Orchiectomy - Removal of a testicle.

Orchiopexy - An operation to bring an undescended testicle down into the scrotum.

Orchitis - Infection in a testicle.

PSA (prostatic specific antigen) - A chemical made by the prostate and released into the blood. PSA levels can be measured. A high PSA may indicate prostate cancer, but

PSA can also be high in patients with BPH and prostatitis. And prostate cancer sometimes occurs in patients with low PSA levels.

Paraphimosis - A condition in which the foreskin has been retracted to expose the glans penis and left in that position. The swollen foreskin makes it difficult to pull the foreskin back over the glans.

Penile-brachial index - A comparison of blood pressure in the penis to blood pressure in the arm. Low blood pressure in the penis as compared to the arm may indicate a problem with blood flow to the penis.

Penile prosthesis - An artificial rod placed in the erectile chambers (corpora) in men with impotency to give the penis rigidity for sex. Penile prostheses are either solid rods that bend or are inflatable.

Performance anxiety - Self-induced stress in a man who is anxious about his sexual performance. The anxiety often makes the erection worse, thus causing more performance anxiety.

Perineal (or perineum) - The area between the scrotum and anus. Men with prostatitis often have pain in the perineum.

Phimosis - A condition in which the foreskin tightens and therefore can't be pulled back to expose the head (glans) of the penis.

Pituitary gland - The gland in the head that makes hormones such as FSH and LH. It is controlled by the hypothalamus but also gets feedback from the testicle which tells it to slow down or speed up the release of FSH and LH.

Plaque (Peyronie's plaque) - Scarring of the penis that may cause penile pain and curvature. Peyronie's plaques may occur in men with impotency who inject medications into the penis to get erections, or they can develop for no apparent reason.

Post-vasectomy pain syndrome - Pain in the scrotum after a vasectomy. It occurs in about 5 percent of men who have vasectomies, but it usually goes away with conservative management (aspirin, jock strap, etc.).

Priapism - A prolonged erection (usually more than three hours) that is often painful and ultimately may scar the penis if not treated. Though rare, this occurs most often in men who use injection therapy for impotency. Various medications (especially those for psychological problems) and sickle cell disease can cause priapism, and sometimes it occurs for no known reason. A man with priapism should see a physician as soon as possible.

Prolactin - A hormone made by the pituitary gland that stimulates the production of milk in a woman's breast. In men, high prolactin levels may adversely affect the testicles (and cause infertility) and the penis (and cause impotency).

Prostatectomy - Removal of the prostate.

Prostatic massage - Massaging or rubbing the prostate gland during a rectal examination to get fluid. It sometimes is done to look for signs of prostate infection (prostatitis).

Prostatism - Symptoms of BPH, like nocturia, frequency, urgency, and a slow urinary stream.

Prostatitis - An infected prostate.

Radical prostatectomy - Surgical removal of the entire prostate gland to treat prostate cancer.

Recanalization - Reconnection of the two cut ends of the vas deferens after a vasectomy.

Reproductive endocrinologist - An obstetrician/gynecologist who has received advanced training in the area of female infertility.

Residual urine - Urine left in the bladder after urination. Usually next to nothing is left in the bladder after urination. Residual urine is common in men with BPH.

Retractile - Refers to a testicle that is retracted or high in the scrotum. This is not considered a problem if it can be pulled manually to the bottom of the scrotum.

Retrograde ejaculation - Ejaculate that goes back into the bladder instead of out the urethra. This is common in men with spinal cord injuries or diabetes and, after the removal of lymph nodes, in men with testicular cancer.

Retrograde semen analysis - Examination of sperm count and motility in the urine of a man with suspected retrograde ejaculation.

Rugae - Wrinkles in the scrotum that develop at puberty.

Scalp reduction - Surgical procedure to remove bald areas of the scalp and increase the percentage of scalp with hair.

Scrotum - The skin that forms the sac containing the testicles.

Secondary sexual characteristics - Characteristics that develop during puberty, including growth of facial, pubic and body hair, a deepening voice, and the growth of muscles.

Semen - Fluid that comes out with ejaculation. Most semen is made by the seminal vesicle followed by the prostate. Sperm makes up only a small amount of semen.

Semen analysis - Examination of semen (an ejaculate) primarily for count, movement, and shape of sperm.

Seminal vesicles - Winglike structures behind the bladder that connect with the vas deferens and contribute the majority of fluid to an ejaculate.

Seminiferous tubules - Long, tiny tubes within the testicle. Sperm (germ cells) develop inside the seminiferous tubules. The most immature germ cells start at the outside of the tubule. As sperm develop, they move towards the center of the tubule where there is an opening for release.

Sertoli cells - Cells in the seminiferous tubules within the testicle. Sertoli cells give support to sperm (germ cells), which are embedded within the Sertoli cells.

Simple prostatectomy - Surgical removal of the enlarged or BPH part of the prostate. This is done when the enlarged part of the prostate is too big to remove by TURP or by one of the new methods of treating BPH, such as microwave therapy. Some prostatic tissue remains after a simple prostatectomy, so prostate cancer may still occur.

Smega - A pasty white collection of sloughed skin and bacteria behind the foreskin.

Spermatid - Sperm developed from a spermatocyte. A spermatid starts as a round cell that looks much like a white blood cell. It develops further by elongating and growing a tail. A mature spermatid is close to being released into the lumen of the seminiferous tubule.

Spermatocyte - A developing sperm that is more mature than a spermatogonia, but less mature than a spermatid.

Spermatogenisis - The growth and development of sperm.

Spermatogonia - The youngest germ cell (a young sperm). It is farthest from the opening in the seminiferous tubule.

Spermatozoa - Another word for sperm.

Suprapubic - The area above the pubic bone where the bladder is located. Men with prostatitis may have suprapubic pain.

TRUS (transrectal ultrasound) - A small probe placed in the rectum that uses sound waves to examine the prostate. TRUS helps locate cancer in the prostate.

TURP (transurethral resection of the prostate) - Shaving out the enlarged or "swollen" part of the prostate as treatment for BPH. TURP, done through the urethra, is like coring an apple.

Telogen - Resting phase of hair.

Testosterone - A hormone primarily made in the testicles. A small amount is also made in the adrenal glands above the kidneys. Testosterone is necessary for the production of sperm, the development of secondary sexual characteristics such as beard growth, and for maintaining a man's sexual drive (or libido).

Torsion - A twisted testicle that cuts off the blood supply to the testicle.

Tumescence - The swelling of a penis filling with blood. A tumesced penis may or may not be hard.

Tunica albuginea - Leatherlike tissue that surrounds the erectile chambers (corpora).

Varicocele - Dilated veins in the scrotum, often described as a "bag of worms."

Vas deferens - The tube connecting the epididymis to the ejaculatory duct. Sperm must travel through the vas deferens to get into the ejaculate. When they are cut in a vasectomy, no sperm gets into the ejaculate.

Vasoepididymostomy - A vasectomy reversal in which the vas deferens is attached above a blocked epididymis to bypass the blockage.

Vasogram - Procedure in which contrast (dye) is injected into the vas deferens to examine for blockages in the vas.

Vasovasotomy - A vasectomy reversal in which the two cut ends of the vas deferens are reattached.

Venous leak - Blood leaking from the erectile chambers. Men with venous leak often complain of difficulty in keeping firm erections.

Voiding - Urinating.

White blood cells (WBCs) - Cells from the immune system that circulate in blood. White blood cells or WBCs try to keep the body free from cancer and bacteria. Lots of WBCs may indicate an infection.

Y chromosome - The "man's chromosome." Humans have 46 chromosomes, and two of them are called "sex chromosomes." A woman's sex chromosomes are X and X, and a man's sex chromosomes are X and Y. One function of the Y chromosome is to direct sperm production.

Index